Death T]
Perc.....

A Collection of Reader-Submitted Medical Stories

Volume 3

Kerry Hamm

Copyright © 2017
All Rights Reserved.

Disclaimer:

Names, locations, and portions of the details included in this book have been altered to protect the privacy of those involved.

By now, I am sure you are all too familiar with my *Real Stories from a Small-Town ER* series, which were collections of stories told to you from my time as a registration clerk in Ohio. If you are new here, don't fret! You don't have to worry about a 'certain order' for *any* of my books, including this one!

I have since moved on from the hospital scene for the time being, but that hasn't stopped readers from submitting stories of their own experiences from the medical field. Since I began writing these books, I have received hundreds of stories-some funny, some sad, some downright scary or grotesque-and have worked with my readers to bring these stories to you in a follow up to my last *Real Stories* volume.

If I've learned anything from writing my series and compiling this book, it's that none of us are alone. No matter how many Negative Nancys want to scold us on how 'nothing in this business is funny' (oh, shut up…yes, it is or there wouldn't be an entire genre available for the stories) or how we should all realize that 'these frustrations are part of the job' and should never be discussed, we're all proof that we've seen some pretty serious messed up things out there, right? We have seen the good. We've seen the bad. We've seen the downright vile and disgusting. And then, we've seen the humor in these situations and we've been fortunate enough to share them with one another. There is a certain peace in knowing that as no matter how crazy we feel, we have formed solidarity amongst ourselves, knowing that for every bad day you've had, others have had them too. We have worked through the challenges of getting up and facing another drug seeker, another child abuse case, another young death, and another 'how the heck did that even happen?' moment together. You guys are not alone, and this book reaffirms that.

Several of the stories have been edited to bring you clear-cut and clean versions of tales submitted by loyal readers. I have done my very best to edit out hospital and town names, and in some cases my submitters wished to withhold their initials and other details from publication or requested that I edit stories for grammar/spelling. Some stories have been edited for length and clarity. I fully believe in writing in 'plain language,' as if you were sitting next to me and I'd recall the stories in person.

Though some of the stories in this collection are horrifying, I am glad none of us are alone in what we've witnessed or experienced.

"No Cops"

Our town isn't too large, but it's definitely not a one-horse town. Even though we have a population of over 35,000, you'd be surprised to know how many of us know one another, even if that means 'knowing of' instead of personally knowing someone.

It seemed most of the nurses up on surgical recovery knew of the patient down the hall from my desk. I'd seen his posts on Facebook, usually on these classifieds or the yard sale pages set up on there, of people selling and buying their old stuff. This guy, from time to time, would try to sell things that nobody in their right mind would ever purchase. One time, he was trying to sell sketches he'd drawn on notebook paper. He was selling them for fifty bucks each. And, I'm not knocking artists at all, but this man was no artist. I guess if you considered stick figures art, maybe. Anyway, that's how I knew of the patient. I'm sure I'd seen his name in the arrests section of our newspaper as well.

This man was on our floor because he fell out of a tree while he was drunk. His spleen ruptured when he landed. The patient never said why he was in the tree in the first place; he was unemployed and didn't live in the area in which the injury occurred. He was transferred to our floor after his surgery, and he didn't cause any of us problems. He mostly kept to himself and played on his phone.

We were all sitting around after the RNs did rounds on their whopping three patients, and most of us whipped out our phones to play on, too. I first checked my texts from my husband, who was out of town. Then I checked with my mother to see how my sons were doing in her care. I then went on Facebook and started scrolling through my timeline. A red dot popped up on my screen to notify me that a new post had been made in the classifieds page I follow. We'd all just gotten paid, so I figured I'd see what was new there.

"You guys," I said, as soon as I read the post, "look at this."

The four of us huddled around my phone and laughed.

"He can't be serious," my coworker said.

"Oh, there's a picture attached," I said. I scrolled down just a bit more.

The post read: IN HOSPITAL, NEED TO MOVE ICE BEFORE THEY FIND IT AND REPORT ME. $100. COME TO ROOM 24-B ON SECOND FLOOR. NO COPS!

Under the post was a picture of a small plastic baggie filled with drugs in the patient's hand. We could even make out his name printed on his hospital bracelet.

In addition to creating this post, the patient tagged the hospital as his current location, so his post was showing up on our facility's Facebook profile.

I'd say it was about ten minutes later, if that, that two officers arrived on our floor. Someone from their station had seen the post and reported it.

When the officers went in the room to confront the patient, the man yelled, "I said no cops!"

My coworkers and I couldn't stop laughing.

Yes, the patient was arrested. He even tried to run from the officers, but he fell out of bed and busted his sutures. We had to page a physician to the floor to repair them and an officer then handcuffed one of the patient's wrists to the bed's side rail.

--J.B.
Indiana

Remorse

My last patient of my shift was a tearful female in her thirties. She signed in with a complaint of a headache. I thought it would be an easy way to end the night, because most of the time we'll take these patients and load them up with some pain meds and Zofran to balance out the feeling of nausea associated with the doses of meds. It usually doesn't take too long to have a patient with a headache cleared for discharge.

When I entered the room for the patient's initial screening, she told me she did not need medical treatment. She stated that she did not know where to go. I immediately assumed we were looking at a case of domestic assault. These cases usually take longer to handle, just because we have to get an advocate in from a domestic assault shelter to see the patient, and we usually have to get law enforcement involved. I do not like clocking out during these cases because I cannot sleep if I don't know my patient will be safe upon discharge.

I rubbed my tired eyes and took a seat on the swivel stool in front of where the patient was sitting. I told her the hospital was a 'safe space' and that nobody could hurt her.

She then asked if she would be arrested for reporting a crime.

Not thinking this through, I told her that she would not be arrested for reporting a crime. I regretted my decision as soon as she told me what the crime was.

The patient was involved in a drug deal. She was the buyer. She purchased a large amount of heroin from her longtime dealer. Then, from what the patient told me, she realized that she was in the process of jeopardizing her week-long sobriety, so she wanted to give the drugs to someone who would destroy them, and she wanted to do so without being charged.

This woman explained that she knew she could have thrown the drugs on the ground or even into the river, but she went on to say that if she did that, she knew she would spend the entire night searching for the drugs and she would end up using again. Her last hope was to give the drugs to someone who could be trusted to get rid of them, someone from whom she could not retrieve the drugs.

Of course, when the woman tried to hand off a plastic bag wrapped up in blue rubber bands, I had to step out of the room and notify the police.

At the time, I didn't know whether to feel guilty, amused at the patient's boldness, or feel sad for her. I felt a mix of guilt and sadness.

This patient was trying to get her life together, and I still applaud her for that. It took a lot of guts for her to present a total stranger with a pouch of illegal drugs. It took a lot of bravery for her to stand up to herself and not shoot up.

Subsequently, the police arrived. I thought the patient would be upset, and I guess she was. She was not hysterical, not the way I thought she would be.

Instead, the patient repeated the story to the officers and said she would like them to arrest the dealer, because "that way [she wouldn't] be tempted to go buy from him again"

Much to my surprise, the officers treated the patient kindly. I don't know the laws, but I am guessing the officers broke them because they told the patient they would treat the heroin as if she found it on the street. She gave the officers details of her dealer's location, and then she asked if she could have a cab voucher to get home. She seemed fearful that her dealer would know she turned him/her in, but more so, she seemed relieved that she didn't have the drugs in her possession.

I will never forget that night. We recently saw this patient for a labor check. She has since married, given birth, and said she's been clean for eighteen months.

--R.P.
Illinois

I'm Aware

A patient waiting to be called back came up to the desk about 9,000 times to ask how long the wait was, ask for food, tattle that the kids in the waiting room were cussing, and complain that ABC Family cut part of a movie she loved.

The straw that broke the camel's back was when she came up to complain to me that the hall floor was wet and I 'really needed to do something about it right now, since I wasn't good for anything else.'

After counting to 20 in my head, I explained to the woman that the floor was wet because the janitor had just mopped, and that's why there was a yellow sign in the center of the hall that read 'WET FLOOR.'

--L.W.
Connecticut

A Security Story

I am a member of law enforcement, contracted to the local hospital for security purposes. I am within my rights to act as law enforcement while on duty. Most people around here know law enforcement is present on hospital grounds, and we have noted a drastic drop in violence or public disturbance since we have been contracted, replacing unarmed security guards. I work hoot owls and it is usually quiet.

One night, I was sitting in the office with my partner. We were drinking coffee and watching television, when out of the corner of my eye, I saw a man's face right up against one of our monitors, meaning his face was centimeters from the security camera. We checked the location: the snack shop. My coworker stated he would go check it out, but we waited for a moment.

We saw the man fidget with the camera. It appeared that he was trying to either disable the camera or remove it completely. He gave up at one point and then attempted to break open a vending machine. When that did not work, he crossed the room, stood on a chair, and fidgeted with the other security camera. By viewing him from another angle, we could see the man was attempting to remove the security camera from the wall by attempting to unscrew the camera. He was using the flat piece of a plastic fork to try to do this.

My partner and I watched the man, rather than approach him. We were amused; it was like watching one of those 'dumbest criminal' shows on TV, only it was live. At one point, the man became angry that he could not get the camera off the wall, so he hit it with his fist, which made him unsteady. He fell off the chair. We laughed.

The man gave up after two hours of his futile attempts. He decided to try the vending machine one last time, and when he couldn't get the coin bank to open, he used a chair to smash the glass front. We watched as he stuffed his pockets with miniature bags of cookies and potato chips.

We met the subject in the hall as he was walking toward the building's exit. He did not speak to us, but we did to him.

"Whatcha going to do with eight bags of Chips Ahoy?" my partner asked.

The man remained calm and said he did not know what the officer was talking about. He tried to portray himself as ignorant.

We explained to the man that we knew his pockets were full of snacks. He finally admitted to this and stated the vending machine was broken when he arrived to the snack shop, but that he made a 'bad decision' to steal, when he should have just alerted someone that the machine had been vandalized.

We arrested the subject. He threw a fit the whole time.

This man tried to fight the charges in court, but he didn't have much to say after two hours of security footage of his face right up against the cameras was shown to the judge. I think he was ordered to community service and restitution.

--C.R.
California

Untitled

Dispatch notified us that a woman called in the death of her four-year-old daughter. We were to meet LEOs on scene and evaluate the need for EMS support.

Upon arrival, my partner and I noted the heavy presence of police officers. We also noted the mother was void of emotion as officers were placing her under arrest. Dispatch failed to tell us that the mother also reported that she killed her own child.

We were called to the child's bedroom. When I say 'called,' I mean it more like someone was shrieking. The man's voice was high-pitched and raw and raspy from how hard he yelled for us.

The little girl's bedroom looked much like my daughter's room. There were dolls on the floor in front of her toy box, and there were so many stuffed animals on the bed that I could hardly see the pink pillows behind them.

Sure, there were dirty clothes hanging out of the hamper and some were on the floor, but overall, the child's room was clean.

Right there, at the foot of the toddler bed, was the four-year-old. She was still blue. Handprints around her neck were already bruising and darkening as each second passed. An officer knelt over her and performed CPR.

"There's a pulse," he frantically announced, in between breathing into the girl's mouth. He pumped on her chest. He was crying.

We practically shoved the officer out of the way and my partner carried the child to the truck. We secured her on the gurney and I began BVM ventilation. I called for an officer to climb in with me. The girl's pulse was faint. I instructed the officer to continue BVM while I did chest compressions.

Two patrol cars attempted to escort our bus through town, but it did not make much difference in time due to the fact that it was a time of day when traffic was heavy. Vehicles did not seem to want to pull over, and intersections are always tricky and unsafe; we lose valuable time crossing through intersections because other cars don't seem to care about running red lights or continuing through normally.

The ER was waiting for us. Their whole team went in the patient's room and someone had already called for a helicopter transport. Unfortunately, no matter how large a city is, sometimes a hospital is simply not certified to handle certain cases. In this case, the hospital was not certified in pediatric trauma.

Our patient was still unresponsive when we left the hospital. I overheard an officer saying the child's father was en route; he had been out with the patient's brother, and officers were able to track him down and escort him to the hospital.

We kept in touch with the ER for report. The child remained unresponsive for three days and was placed on life support with little to no chance of recovery due to the amount of time her brain had been deprived of oxygen. Even if she did come to, her quality of life would be drastically different from before the incident; doctors said she would be unable to perform tasks on her own, would be confined to a wheelchair, would likely never talk, and would be severely mentally impaired. On the fourth day, her father made the difficult decision to remove life support.

From what we heard over time, the mother stated she killed her child because she 'felt angry.'

--U.D.
Texas

Man in his thirties was brought in by his friends because he got drunk and taunted a moose. The moose got fed up and charged. The man had to go to surgery for internal bleeding. His BAC was .56.

--E.D.
Alaska

<u>Entitled</u>

We received the call a little after 02:00 that EMS was en route with a critical trauma following an MVA. The vehicle was found totaled in an empty wheat field in the middle of winter. The patient was found without identification, but he was able to give his name and age.

When the patient arrived, it was all hands-on deck in his room. We were looking at internal bleeding in the patient's abdominal region, tachycardia, and a brain bleed, as well as multiple broken bones. Our doctor believed the patient's neck was broken, and unfortunately, he was correct. The patient sustained a broken neck, crushed vertebrae, broke both legs, and bones in both arms were essentially shattered. The patient was in shock and when he could speak, he would scream in agony. Officers requested we did not sedate the patient until they could attempt to gather more information.

Ordinarily, I would demand to know why the officers would request such a thing, but in this case, it was clear: the patient was not the driver of the vehicle. He was found in the passenger seat. The driver of the vehicle was nowhere to be found.

After twenty minutes of questioning the patient and waiting through his cries and shouts, the officers learned the patient's friend had been the driver. Once the officers gathered a name—the only piece of information they were able to gather in that period—they nodded that we could sedate the patient. He was being prepped for emergency flight transfer.

Officers found the patient's friend. He was found staggering a few miles from the initial crash site. Officers almost ran the teenager over because he was walking down the center of a country road in the pitch-black night. EMS brought the driver to us, and he was covered in blood. His BAC was three times the legal limit, and that was considering the legal limit was for someone of drinking age, which he was not.

The driver was cocky and overall rude as all get-out. He seemed to treat the entire situation like a big joke and didn't seem to mind that he was in the center of a big mess. He laughed when an officer stated he was facing charges. The patient was found to also have a broken neck and was placed in a brace. Luckily, that was the only real injury he sustained in the crash, other than superficial lacerations and contusions to his hands and face.

What really got us all riled up about this patient is that not only he admitted to driving under the influence, but he also admitted to leaving his friend there to die. He admitted to taking his friend's wallet and cell phone so the passenger could not call for help. He'd hoped that by taking the passenger's wallet, the passenger would die and therefore nothing would link him (the driver) to the scene, as even the car belonged to the passenger.

This teenager was a hateful person with no soul.

It wasn't over, not yet.

The patient's father arrived and took the charge nurse, doctor, and two officers aside. He was well-known in the community for his wealth and powerful position in politics. He wanted to know 'what could be done' to keep his son's name out of the reports, and he even suggested blaming the situation on another local teenager who'd attended the same party his son and the passenger had attended. He had zero guilt or shame in suggesting someone else be held responsible for his son's actions. He offered monetary rewards in exchange of our staff altering our records, as well as the officers falsifying their records.

The patient's father was arrested for bribery, but the charge didn't stick because he hired lawyers that basically stated all four of the people he had talked to were lying. The patient's son was arrested for leaving the scene of an accident, but he was also released on his attorney's argument that he was 'confused.'

The passenger of the vehicle lived. He did face months of recovery and underwent multiple surgeries. We don't know what happened to the driver, but his father is still involved in local politics and his lifestyle doesn't seem to have been affected by his son's actions whatsoever.

    --K.L.
    Iowa

Just Desserts

I hadn't been at work for a whole two minutes before Charge gave me my first patient. I had a few minutes to prepare, but I was admittedly puzzled over why a patient with a testicular injury was arriving via EMS with law enforcement tailing.

We could all hear the patient before he was even in the building. He was a young thing, just hanging on to his teen years. He was sobbing and doubled over on the stretcher when he was transported inside. The crotch of his mesh shorts was bloody and something was hanging out of the leg of the patient's shorts.

That something was his scrotum.

Good grief! What could possibly have occurred to sustain this sort of injury?

The patient, being a jackass as he tried to show off to friends while they were visiting a petting zoo, decided to punch a Shetland pony. In return, the pony (which we found out later was named Kick) kicked the patient in the testicles, which busted the scrotum. The patient lost the innards of his left portion of his scrotum.

As if this wasn't bad enough, the whole thing was recorded because the patient wanted a 'funny' video to post on his Facebook timeline.

And the patient was arrested for felony animal abuse.

--A.C.
Wyoming

<u>Here Comes Peter Cottontail</u>

The strangest patient I'd ever had to clear for a jail clearance was a woman who was arrested for chasing children down the block of a subdivision. Our town is small, and I can honestly say we've never quite had this problem before, but alcohol and bath salts aren't a great combination.

What was so strange about this patient was that she was dressed in a bunny costume. I don't mean she was dressed as a sexy rabbit, like a Playboy bunny with sexy tights and a bra as a top. She wasn't even dressed as a scary rabbit. This costume was basically a fluffy white onesie with huge pink bunny ears on the hood.

I couldn't stop laughing during the assessment and clearance because all I could imagine was this grown woman wearing a bunny costume chasing screaming kids down the street in the middle of June.

The patient was booked for disorderly conduct, public intoxication, and disturbing the peace.

--B.R.
Colorado

Madness

I was a one of the responding medics dispatched to a sorority mixer hosted at a local museum dedicated to our community's history. Our history is rich in fishing, has a Coast Guard base that was initially started as a local team who responded to maritime distress, and our town is known for a famous Mom and Pop diner. The artifacts in the museum reflect that history. There are buoys from the original distress team's business, as well as a giant plaster bust of the diner's mascot.

The scene was a crap-show, it really was. There were cops all over the place, and all these sorority chicks and fraternity guys were running all over the place. There were pools of vomit on the carpet. The mixer took place in the museum's banquet room, but the crowd had taken the party to the halls of the museum and artifacts had become damaged. Someone had taken a pair of panties and placed them on the plaster mascot's head. There were lipstick drawings on the glass cases of many artifacts, and some of the cases had been broken, with the contents missing. I spotted on girl passed out on the floor. She was wearing a pair of diving goggles she'd stolen from the museum. People were being tased and handcuffed and pepper sprayed. The curator of the museum was called in and he was screaming and weeping because of all the damage. He seemed more upset about the artifacts being damaged than he did about the condition of the building. I witnessed both men and women urinating on the floors and on the museum artifacts.

Our patient was in the bathroom, holding what appeared to be an entire roll of unraveled paper towels to the back of his head. His girlfriend was crying and vomiting into the toilet. The young stud said the two were trying to have sex in the bathroom, but when he sat on the sink's edge, the sink broke loose from the wall and he hit his head.

Some of the other medics on scene were transporting patients for high BACs, and one team transported a patient who was shot in the leg by one of the harpoons the museum had on display.

I heard the sorority was sued for damages that exceeded $40,000.

--B.W.
South Carolina

Too Much Eggnog

I was patrolling and saw a man with an axe on the courthouse lawn. I called in my location to dispatch and requested assistance in case I needed it.

"Sir," I said, "can you tell me what you're doing?"

He pointed to the this forty-foot Evergreen and said in a slur, "I need a Christmas tree."

I said to the man, "Sir, are you aware you're standing on the lawn of the courthouse?"

He looked around and then shrugged. "A tree can't *belong* to anyone but God."

"Is this something you think you should be doing right now?" I asked. "What made you decide to do this?"

I about died when the guy told me, "Well, I've had a bunch to drink."

The man took another swing at the base of the tree, where he'd barely made a dent, and when he drew the axe back, he smacked himself in the face with the butt, cracking the bridge of his nose open.

Medics transported the man to the ER after I read him his rights, and he was booked on public intox. We let everything else slide.

After a night in the drunk tank (with a bandage across his face), the man said he was embarrassed and that he didn't even know how he thought he was going to get the tree moved or in his house, seeing that he walked to the courthouse and lived in a mobile home that certainly did not have a forty-foot ceiling.

--J.U.
Kentucky

Roadkill

My partner and I were dispatched to an MVA just off the highway. We were informed fire rescue would arrive shortly, as there were reports from multiple callers that the driver was trapped in the vehicle.

Indeed, once we arrived on scene, we noted the patient was trapped inside. Her vehicle had rolled several times before resting in a deep ditch. It was impossible to open her door, and the passenger's door was smashed against the ground. Yes, her car was resting in a sideways position.

The patient, still buckled, was screaming.

We yelled through the window for her to calm down, that fire rescue would arrive shortly and would use their machinery to extract the patient from her vehicle. She continued screaming.

It took fifteen minutes for the fire team to remove the patient's car door, during which time she continued screaming.

"Get me out!" she ordered us. "Hurry! It's biting me!"

Okay. So, if someone told you this, wouldn't you think that person was high on drugs? That's what I was thinking, until I moved in closer and could hardly breathe from the stench of alcohol emitting from the woman's car and breath.

"It's biting me!" she repeated.

"Ma'am," I said, "please remain calm. We're doing all we can to remove you safely."

I reached around the woman's body to hold her up as my partner cut the seatbelt from her, and that's when I felt a sharp pain to my finger. I jerked away just as my partner cut the belt, so the patient toppled over and then started cursing because she said I dropped her on purpose.

I examined my finger. The latex glove was torn and I was bleeding.

Before I had a chance to even guess what had occurred, this gigantic opossum waddled out from behind the driver's seat and just walked between my partner and me. My partner screamed and jumped out of the way.

"I told you it was biting me!" the patient shouted at me.

"Why was there a opossum in your car?" I shouted back.

"I thought it was dead!" the woman yelled, which left me even more confused.

The woman hit the animal, stopped, put it in her car, and had every intention of taking the animal home, where she planned to bury it…not because she felt sorry, but because she 'didn't want to get arrested for murder.'

She was instead arrested for drunk driving. She and I were both treated to a series of injections, just in case the animal had rabies.

--I.P.
Alabama

Abuse of Power

Many years ago, I worked at a nursing home and some of the nurses there were hateful to the residents. I learned from that place to listen to family members, even if what they say sounds absurd.

One nurse went to a man's room and told him his wife and son had been killed in a car accident. She told the man that wife had been driving and she veered into oncoming traffic, where her vehicle was hit head-on by a semi. The patient was distraught and had a heart attack after hearing this false news.

Another patient was known as a violent troublemaker during her stay. Because she was known to be violent, she was kept restrained and/or sedated. She was known for throwing her belongings about the room. We'd often be responsible for picking up broken porcelain picture frames and glass, clothing, shoes—you name it—after one of her episodes.

This turned out to be a lie, too. The woman's great-granddaughter thought something felt 'wrong,' so she hid a teddy bear camera in the patient's room. It turns out one of the nurses was the one destroying the patient's room, simply because she thought it was 'funny.'

My final straw at that place was learning some of the nurses were stealing and pocketing patient medication. Several of us filed formal complaints that were finally taken seriously. The nurses involved in all these complaints were fired, and some of them faced charges.

Not all nursing homes are like this, but I really learned to listen to patients instead of brushing off their stories as 'tall tales.'

--N.P.
Oklahoma

I once saw a patient come in for a finger trauma. He said he stuck his index finger between the blades of a new pair of tree pruning shears because he 'wanted to see' if they were sharp enough to cut through bone.

They were.

He lost his finger.

--S.T.
Indiana

__Goin' Through the Big D__

Everyone in our tiny town knew John and Jane were getting divorced. Even without all the gossip, it was pretty big news to miss because they always had us out to moderate arguments that had turned to full-blown fistfights in the yard between John and Jane's new beau, Jim. Jim, at one point, was John's best friend and still was his business partner. The two started up an excavation company and were doing pretty well for themselves. Jane kicked John out of their new manufactured doublewide and moved Jim in. John rented a trailer on the other side of town, which around here, means he ended up a few blocks away.

In the beginning days of the divorce process, John would drink and make harassing phone calls to Jane. Within a month's time, this escalated into John going to his previous home. The first time we picked him up, he and Jim were throwing punches in the front yard and the sliding glass door to the home was shattered. Both men were taken to the local hospital to be stitched up and then were taken to jail. We held them overnight but charges were dropped because we figured the men were just too hotheaded from everything going on.

Over the next few weeks, our station received no fewer than twenty calls from John, Jane, or Jim. They behaved like toddlers, tattling on each other for every little thing. Jane wanted us to know John's truck registration was expired. John wanted us to do something about Jane swiping a ten-dollar-bill from church offering two years ago. Jim wanted to let us know John was the one who stole that cattle crossing sign last year. I probably answered half of those calls. The sheriff stepped in and put his foot down. He personally called all three back and told them to stay away from each other, stop calling each other, and most importantly—stop calling our station unless it was an emergency, as in someone had been shot or was having a heart attack.

Jim quit the excavation partnership and took John to court to receive half of the business. Jane was trying to get the house, all the vehicles, half of John's portion of his business, and had a list of demands so long that it would stretch across the state.

Unexpectedly, John agreed to hand over his *entire* business to Jim and Jane. He signed over two dozers and two track hoes. They were supposed to meet at the courthouse on a Friday to sign all the paperwork. John's only request in all of this is that he would receive twenty-percent of the business profits for a year. We all thought he was nuts.

You'd think the fighting would be over because of this, but Jane still wasn't happy. We were called out a few days before John and Jim's court date because the three were all at the bar and John and Jim were fighting again. We locked them up for the night again.

Everything was quiet the next day. John and Jim appeared to have come to terms with everything and were laughing and joshing around when we released them. It was great to see them back on good terms, just like before all this mess had started. Someone asked John what changed his mind and he said he was tired of all the fighting.

That night, the sheriff called me at home and told me to meet him over at Jane's. I was hotter than a coal in a barbeque because I was just settling in for the evening. No sooner than I hung up the phone, however, I heard sirens whooping. Our town's two fire trucks sped out from the station across the street from my house.

(The reader's initial reaction to this moment was omitted due to an attempt to keep this version 'clean.' Imagine a great deal of cussing.)

When I had arrived, John was in cuffs and Jane was crying into Jim's shoulder. She and Jim had come back from a steak dinner at the Moose club to find the doublewide aflame and John sitting in a folding lawn chair in the gravel driveway.

John had told Jane (which even John proudly admitted to saying), "Why stop at taking half of everything? You can have my half of the ashes. Take it all, Jane!"

Oh, boy.

Not only did John burn down Jane's trailer, but he also took every last piece of machinery from his business and sank them all in the river. It took four days to tow it all out because we had to call in a crew from the city.

Jane and Jim ended up getting married while John was in prison.

--R.B.
Texas

A man came in with severe facial trauma—he sustained an orbital fracture, broken nose, and was missing two teeth.

When we asked the police officer standing outside the room what had happened, he said the man was trying to slash his girlfriend's tires, but he didn't do it correctly and the tire exploded in his face.

To make matters worse, the car didn't even belong to the man's girlfriend; he targeted the wrong car in a fast food parking lot.

--D.W.
Oregon

<u>Help Me, I'm Dead</u>

Here's a real conversation I had with a patient, after the registration clerk called me to deal with him.

Me: What seems to be the problem today, sir?

Patient: I stopped breathing an hour ago.

Me: Do you have a history of breathing issues? Have you been diagnosed with asthma or anything of the sort?

Patient: No.

Me: How long would you guess you went without breath?

Patient: *He looks at me like I'm stupid.* An hour. I just told you.

Me: You said you stopped breathing an hour ago. But, I mean, how long were you without breath? Thirty seconds? Five seconds?

Patient: *Clearly agitated* An hour. I stopped breathing an hour ago.

Me:

Patient: I never started breathing again.

Me: Sir, if you weren't breathing, you wouldn't be able to talk to me right now, and you certainly wouldn't be standing in the lobby unassisted.

Patient: *The man dramatically falls to the floor.* Help me. I haven't taken a breath in an hour.

Me:

Registration: What is he doing?

Me: I don't know.

Patient: Not breathing, that's for sure.

Me: Sir, please stand up.

Patient: Help me. I'm not breathing.

Me: If you weren't breathing, you would be dead right now, as in not talking, not squirming around, and not doing much of anything.

Patient: *Stops talking for ten seconds, then turns head to face the next shift of nurses coming on duty.* Help me. I stopped breathing and I'm dead.

Me, to registration: Call a counselor.

Patient: Don't call a counselor. Call the morgue.

The patient tested positive for meth. I can't say I was a bit surprised on that one.

--E.D.
Kentucky

But I Have a Permit

We don't allow weapons on hospital grounds. We even have a sign in the lobby that says if you are carrying a knife or weapon, that you either lock it in your vehicle or log it with our security department. When you leave the hospital, you can sign a ticket from security and they will give you back your weapon. For the most part, this has worked. Our people are usually easy going and we're all from the country, so we know how to keep the peace and understand the rules.

This one night, a guy came in because he said his leg hurt. I finished registering him and a nurse called him over to an exam room. That's when she saw the man was carrying a pistol in a side holster. She pointed to the sign by the entrance and told the man he either had to take his gun to his vehicle, or he had to log it with our security department. He told her he couldn't take it to his vehicle because his mom dropped him off, and then he said he wouldn't log it with security because he had every right to carry it.

When the nurse said that she would not escort the man to the exam room if he was armed, the guy flipped out and started yelling that he had a concealed carry permit and was allowed to have the gun with him if he wanted to do so. We told him we know most of the people in our area are armed and we weren't against that, but at the hospital we needed to provide a safe environment for our patients and staff. He was being belligerent so I called the security department and asked the officers to come to the ER lobby.

This only made everything worse.

The man refused to hand over his gun. He also refused to leave. Those were his only options. We all tried to explain to the man that disarming patients and/or visitors was in everyone's best interest, but he continued to argue.

That's when the man pulled his pistol from his holster and held it up. He was waving it around and security told me to call 911 and activate a code to keep everyone away from the ER due to someone with a weapon.

"I'm not going to shoot anyone," the man said. "I know how to use a gun. I have a permit. I'm safe. I'm one of the good guys."

He pointed the pistol at me and I freaked out and screamed. Then he pointed it at the security guards. He was laughing and said not to worry, that he knew what he was doing.

He then pointed it at his foot and said, "It can't even do anything. The safety's on."

He pulled the trigger and the gun went off.

Yep, Mr. Safety shot himself in the foot.

At least he was in the emergency room when he did it.

The man was cited for discharging his weapon in public.

--S.K.
Tennessee

Canned Karma

I'm a medic. The owner of our company got this bright idea to put a pop machine across the street from our station. He said if we were thirsty to go across the street and buy a soda. I think it was just another way for him to make money off us and everyone in town, but none of us even use that machine. The only people I've ever seen use it have been kids walking across town or people you know have drug and alcohol problems.

One night, we were having a cookout in the parking lot, when we saw this guy walk up to the pop machine and start messing with the coin slot. He wasn't trying to get a pop. He was trying to break into it to steal the money and probably thought he could stash a few pops in his pants pockets, too. He didn't care at all that cars were driving by or that we were all outside watching him.

The man tried to pry the coin bank off with a screwdriver, but the tool bounced back and the man stabbed himself in the upper shoulder. He cussed and was bleeding, but he brushed it off.

Then, even after failing, the man started to kick the machine and grabbed it and was rocking it back and forth. We thought for sure he was going to pull the thing down on himself, but he didn't.

Angry that his master plan wasn't working, the man made a fist with the screwdriver still in his hand. He hit the front of the machine with his knuckles and his hand bounced off. He screamed when he stabbed himself again with the screwdriver, this time in his pec.

The man was now bleeding in two spots and was screaming that his hand hurt. He turned around and yelled to us that he needed someone to take him to the hospital, but we can't do anything unless someone calls in to dispatch.

So, the man walked across the street and asked to use one of our cell phones. He called

911 and dispatch actually sent us across the street to take this guy to the ER.

The man ended up getting a few stitches for his stab wounds, had his broken hand wrapped up, and then his nurse called the police because he admitted he had been attempting to commit a crime. The cops laughed and said it served the man right to get stabbed. Then they arrested him because he had a crack pipe on him and had warrants.

Our boss was afraid someone else would do something like that and he'd get sued, so he made this wire cage thing to encase the pop machine. Nobody's been able to break into it yet.

    --R.F.
    Ohio

Gotta Go, Gotta Go, Gotta Go Right Now

The registration guy had to run papers to another department, so he asked me to sit at the front desk in case any patients arrived. I'm an RN and don't know how to sign people in, so I was a little nervous, but figured the clerk in back could sign someone in if they came in for treatment.

I stared off into space for a few minutes, before a peculiar man in the waiting room caught my attention. He appeared antsy and agitated. I assumed he was a family member or friend of a drug overdose in one of our treatment rooms. He caught me looking at him and screamed something, so I looked away and began flipping through a sporting catalog the registration guy had at his desk.

Just a few seconds later, I heard a grumble from the end of the hallway. I looked up to see the agitated man from the waiting room was trying to get in the restroom.

He kept pulling on the door that was supposed to be pushed. When he couldn't get in the restroom, he used his fist to bang on the door.

"Sir," I called.

He yelled at me to shut up, so I decided not to tell him that he was pulling instead of pushing.

The man continued banging on the door and shouting for the occupant to hurry up.

After another two minutes of this, I called down to him again. "Sir?"

He called me a name and told me to mind my business. I called our overnight janitor and asked him to come to the department to handle an agitated gentleman.

Before the janitor arrived to either calm the gentleman or escort him from the department, the man picked up a no-smoking sign and swung it at the door. The top piece of the sign fell to the floor, while the metal bar to which it was attached ricocheted off the door and hit the man in the nose. He fell to the ground like a tin can shot with a bb gun.

This angry, mean-spirited young man effectively knocked himself out cold because he couldn't be bothered to take two seconds to listen to that 'crotchety old hag' at the registration desk.

I still think it serves him right.

--W.J.
South Dakota

Real 911 call:

A mother called after her child had been sent home from school for having lice. She told me the girl must have gotten it from school and she wanted an officer to come out so she could press charges.

--S.D.
Florida

Just Go Home

The most frustrating patient I've ever dealt with was this girl who was in her first semester at university. Like your hospital, these college kids come in with all 900 of their friends for the most asinine reasons, and all 900 of those friends act like it's the end of the world for their friend.

This girl came in with at least 10 friends and they were all whooping and hollering in the waiting room as they watched a basketball game on the overhead television.

"What seems to be the problem tonight?" I asked her.

She handed me a bottle of Tylenol and said, "I took some of these and forgot I was allergic."

"What kind of reaction do you usually have when you take these?"

She shrugged. "I don't know. I don't take them."

"What kind of reaction are you having right now?"

She looked at me like I was stupid and said, "I'm not, but I'm allergic."

I sighed and asked how many she took. She told me she took one or two, that she couldn't remember.

"What do you mean, you can't remember?" I asked.

She explained, "Well, I didn't take them tonight. I took them yesterday and just realized today that I took them."

I kind of stared at her.

"Did you have a reaction yesterday?" I asked.

She shook her head.

When I tried to explain to the girl that she did not need to be in the emergency room almost midnight for medication she took the day before, she started screaming at me and telling me I didn't know what I was talking about because I'm not a nurse or a doctor.

So, you know what I did? I called the doctor away from his desk and asked him to come up and explain the same thing to the girl.

The doctor laughed when the girl told him everything she had just told me. He informed her she either was not allergic to that medicine, or she did not take enough to set off an allergic reaction. She argued with him and demanded to be seen.

That girl ended up with a $1,200 bill from the emergency room just because she couldn't use common sense.

--T.W.
Arizona

One of my patients told me she thought she had gonorrhea and wanted me to test for it.

I am her dentist.

--H.S.
Washington

Throw Stones

Me, an M.D. at a suburban ER: Ms. Smith, your chart says you're experiencing vaginal irritation, burning, and discharge. Is that correct?

Ms. Smith: Yeah. I think I have chlamydia again.

Me: Again?

Ms. Smith: Yeah. I get it every few months. It's real annoying, ya know?

Me: We can most certainly test for that and prescribe an antibiotic. You know, the safest way to protect yourself is to always use a condom during intercourse and have yourself tested regularly if you believe your partner may be infected.

Ms. Smith: *Grumbles something about how she knows this.*

I started a vaginal exam on Ms. Smith, only to find a foreign object shoved inside her vaginal cavity.

Me: It, uh, seems that you have something inside of your body.

Ms. Smith: Oh, yeah. I bought these healing stones off Ebay. It said they're supposed to, like, absorb all the bad stuff from your body. Supposed to, like, rub them over your arms if they hurt and stuff.

This 'healing stone' was one of those shimmering rocks that homeowners use for landscaping.

--J.P.
Pennsylvania

Mental Instability

I am not one to mock the mentally ill, but one patient will always be burned in my memories.

Mr. Smith barely walked himself through the ER doors. He collapsed just inside the lobby, and the check-in girl called me to come up to help. She neglected to tell me Mr. Smith was bleeding out.

I called out for someone to get a gurney, and my coworkers and I, with the help of our security team, lifted the Mr. Smith to the gurney and rushed him straight back. It was not immediately known what had happened, but Mr. Smith's t-shirt was soaked in blood, as were his sweatpants.

In a trauma room, we cut Mr. Smith's clothes from his body. He was hardly conscious. He kept trying to talk to us, but we repeatedly informed him to stay quiet and calm, as panicking would only make it worse. We did not want him to arrest.

It became clear that Mr. Smith had taken a sharp object and sliced open his abdomen. The laceration was deep and extended across his whole abdomen.

He refused to remain still and repeatedly pulled the oxygen mask from his mouth. Mr. Smith grabbed a nurse by the arm and asked, "Can you save the baby?"

This man fully believed he was pregnant and he 'performed a C-section' on himself because he thought he was in labor and later stated nobody believed that he was pregnant.

Mr. Smith was transferred to our psychiatric unit effective immediately following his surgery. He was transferred back to the ER for multiple suicide attempts in the short time he was on the floor because he thought the nurses stole his child and this caused him to fall in a great depression stage.

One of our mental health counselors gave Mr. Smith a baby doll her daughter had outgrown, and Mr. Smith calmed down enough to heal from his surgery and suicide attempts. He was then transferred to an assisted living facility for the mentally unstable.

--T.R.
New Hampshire

One sure-fire way to go to jail: My guy handed me an ID at a traffic stop, but then asked for it back because 'I accidentally gave you the fake one, man.'

He handed me his *real* ID, the one that said he was under 21 and wasn't of age to be drinking the vodka from the bottle he had resting between his legs.

--J.B.
Rhode Island

So THAT is What You Meant!

I, too, work in the ER as a registration assistant. My most memorable stupid person came in during a rush and he waited in line for almost fifteen minutes.

"How can I help you, sir?" I asked.

"My wife cut her hand and it's bleeding bad. There's blood everywhere."

"Let's get her registered, then," I said.

The man gave me his wife's name, date of birth, social, address, and just about everything else we needed. I was excited that he knew all of her information and that he had his insurance cards handy because it would save me from having to pull him in the billing booth later.

"If you want to get your wife and bring her in, we can have a nurse assess her injury and see if we can get her back a little sooner," I said.

He looked dumbstruck.

"Uh, she's not here."

She's not here? She's not here? What does he mean that she's not here? I just registered her and everything. She was now in our system, and this guy is telling me she's not here?

"What do you mean?" I asked, trying to calm my inner self.

"She's at home."

"She's at home?"

He nodded.

"If she's bleeding, why did you come to the hospital without her?"

"Because she didn't say she was coming."

I was so lost.

"What?"

The man said, "Our phones are out of minutes. She told me to go get help."

We called 911 from the registration department and an ambulance transported the man's wife to the ER.

"I told you to get help!"

He yelled back, "I did!"

And then the lady screamed, "I meant for you to go to the neighbor's house to use the phone, idiot!"

"Well, you didn't say that! You just said to go get help!"

The lady yelled, "I just assumed you would have enough sense not to drive across town to the hospital, stupid!"

The kicker to all of this was that the doctor used the husband's cell phone and showed him that even though the plan was out of minutes, the couple could have still called 911 because cell phones are capable of dialing for emergencies.

--P.B.
New Jersey

Give the Dog a Bone

My boss: Jane, Mrs. Smith filed a formal complaint against you because she said you refused her service while she was in the ER.

Me, confused: But she was seen in the ER, so…?

My boss: She said you refused her service.

Me, remembering Mrs. Smith's visit: Oh, she was mad because we didn't have a jar of treats so she could give one to her dog. I told her this is a hospital and we don't keep dog treats here. Then she got mad, called me a name, and left.

My boss, shaking her head: Never mind. I'll take care of the complaint.

--M.S.
Missouri

Hot Shot

Since I work the overnight shift, I don't tend to have much free time to run errands. Before my shift, which starts at midnight, I usually run to the grocery store for pre-packaged food to take as 'lunch.' In all the time I've been doing this, I've only had one problem, and it was the scariest experience of my life.

I stopped at the store with a list in mind. I distinctly remember I wanted to get some of those frozen PB & J sandwich bites, and then I wanted to get a few drinks and a small bag of chips. I also needed to grab something for the carry in, so I was going to stop by the bakery section on the way to the checkout counter and see about buying a small cake.

Halfway through the store, I realized I didn't have enough cash on me. I couldn't use my debit card because for some reason it wouldn't swipe in that grocery store, so while

I was waiting for a replacement to come in the mail, I had been withdrawing cash from the ATM to do my grocery shopping.

The ATM at this grocery store was located outside, probably close to fifteen feet from their entrance. I walked outside with no fear because nothing had ever happened to me before, so I guess I didn't think anything would happen to me then.

A man saw me, some single woman in scrubs, as a target, and I heard him before I saw him. He shoved something sharp against the small of my back and told me to hand him my money as it was sliding out of the dispenser.

I was stupid and told him, "But it's only twenty dollars."

He grabbed my arm so hard I thought the skin was going to tear. He spun me around and I realized I didn't have much of a chance of physically fighting back because he was at least two feet taller than I was and he was exceptionally fit.

This man punched me in the face and I defensively shoved him away. That's when he stabbed me. I didn't know if it was on purpose or if the box cutter slipped during the altercation. I remember thinking at the time that he appeared mighty surprised that I was bleeding from my side.

Within a split second, I recalled there was pepper spray in my purse. I doubled over and reached to the bottom of my bag until I felt the container. I couldn't stand up all the way because my wound felt like it was stretching open and every centimeter I moved caused more blood to soak through my scrubs. The blood was seeping down my side and ran down my pants.

I sprayed the man dead in the face with pepper spray and he screamed. I started yelling for help and tried to run back to the store. When I turned back to make sure the man was not following me, I saw he was running away. He wasn't running in a straight line, but he was running nonetheless.

One of the overnight stockers came outside for a smoke break and saw that I was bleeding. He called 911 and I passed out before the ambulance arrived. I was transported to the local ER, where I tech.. It was an odd feeling to be a patient, rather than tend to one.

The doctor said my wound was deep, but it was nothing that sutures and time couldn't fix. He prepped me to receive twenty-two stitches. I never realized that the man who attacked me dragged the box cutter. I only thought I had one small puncture wound.

As I was being prepped for sutures, I heard my assailant's voice from the hallway. I was so afraid that I nearly fell out of bed. I told the doctor the voice I heard was that of the man who'd just attacked me. The doctor asked if I was absolutely certain, of which I was. I will never forget that man's voice.

My coworkers were assisting the man through the ER. He was coughing and threw up on the floor before he reached his room. He was still in the clothes he was wearing when he assaulted me. I heard through chatter that he told his nurse that he was mugged and pepper sprayed, and now he was not only experiencing the normal side effects of the spray, but he was also allergic to something in it. The man could hardly breathe and his face looked like a cartoon character's.

My doctor called the police while the man's nurse called as well. Officers took both statements. I felt like they thought I was lying because they made me tell my story three times. Finally, I handed one of the officers my container of pepper spray and told him the bottle said that the spray was UV sensitive, meaning it would show up under a UV light to prove it was my spray on the man's face. All that time, the man had no idea that I was in the same emergency room. I doubt he would have even cared, since he obviously did not care enough about my life in the first place.

After the man was medically cleared, he was arrested on suspicion of bodily harm and robbery with a weapon or something like that. I was incredibly disappointed to learn he was released due to a technicality. Just a few weeks later, though, I saw he had been arrested for home invasion, drug possession, assault with a deadly weapon, illegal firearm possession, and intent to deal. He was sentenced to prison.

I still go to that grocery store before work, but I make sure I am alert when I am in the parking lot. I do not travel without my pepper spray, and I also bought a stun gun to keep in my purse. I carry that when I am walking in and out of the store at night.

--P.F.
Delaware

Busted

    Where I work, the uppers give out an award each month that is the equivalent to Employee of the Month. If you win, you get a decent bonus in your paycheck, get a bunch of coupons and vouchers for food places and businesses around town, and you get a designated parking spot in your assigned parking lot, which is probably the best part of the deal because ordinarily we must park at least a block away from the building. That rarely means we park a block away because there's never a spot open, so most of us end up in the parking garage and walk almost three blocks to even get in our main building. Imagine doing this in the rain or snow a few times a month, and you can see why someone would want that reward.

    Because the rewards are so 'lucrative,' many of the employees are highly competitive against one another. They're always trying to outdo each other on getting the highest numbers or most reports or treating patients over-the-top nicely so they can hopefully get the patients to either call or write back on a comment card. Each call or comment card helps you in the running for the monthly award.

This guy in Lab was so angry that he didn't get the award, that he went off the deep end.

The day after another man in Lab was awarded Employee of the Month, the first man keyed the winner's car and slashed his tires. We didn't know it was the sore loser who did that at first.

I came in for my shift one morning and the police were down the hall, questioning the Lab loser. I could tell it was a big deal because our security guys were there, as well as the head of the hospital, two nursing supervisors, and the man's boss. The man was arrested right there. I hurried back to my department because I didn't want to get in trouble for snooping, even though everyone else in that area was staring.

The sore loser had been stealing hospital equipment from the CS department. He started selling crutches, boots, and sterilized tools on Craigslist and even had a few posts of the items on Facebook. Someone from the hospital saw one of the man's posts on Facebook and recognized the packaged sterilized tool as something that was never meant to leave hospital grounds. The packaging even had our hospital name on it!

When the man was questioned, he admitted to vandalizing the winner's car, and he expressed his frustrations of not winning the monthly award. Before he was handcuffed and escorted off hospital property, the head of the hospital told the man he had never received the award because of his bad attitude.

I could definitely see that.

--O.C.
Michigan

Time is a Tricky Thing

Oh my good heavens, I laughed so hard at your time zone story because I've had a similar experience.

I work with orders, and they come from all over the country because we are a top-rated facility and are well-known in the USA for what we can offer patients.

A call came through and I answered. The woman on the line stated she was from a doctor's office in California. She stated that three minutes ago she sent an order through our online services and wanted to make sure that we received it.

"I'm sorry, Ma'am," I said, "but a new order from your practice is not registering in my system as of yet. It usually takes between ten and fifteen minutes for new orders to show on my end."

"But you're two hours ahead of us."

"I'm sorry?"

"You're two hours ahead."

"Sorry, but that's not how this works," I stated.

The woman began shouting at me. She screamed, "What are you not understanding about this? I just sent it. If you are two hours ahead of us, that means you would have gotten the order almost two hours ago."

"Ma'am," I said, trying not to laugh at how crazy she was sounding.

"Don't interrupt me. And don't try to give me some excuse," she told me. "Why is none of this making sense to your pea-brain? Give me your supervisor now."

"There are these invisible things called 'time zones,' Ma'am," I stated to the caller.

She was still angry and demanded to know the time in my office.

"It's 8:32."

"Well," she hissed, "I sent that form through the computer at 6:23. So why haven't you gotten it?"

"Ma'am," I said again, "there are time zones."

"But it's been two hours! You should have gotten it already! I don't even know how you guys are in business with how stupid you people are."

She refused to talk to me further and ordered that I transfer her to my supervisor. The supervisor informed the receptionist that he was recording the woman's rant, to which she replied that she didn't care because she knew she was right.

I received a phone call from the owner of the practice a few hours later. The doctor apologized to me a thousand times for how his receptionist had treated me, and he said she was no longer with his practice.

--P.I.

Location withheld at request

<u>Just the Nips, Ma'am</u>

On Easter weekend, LEOs brought in two strippers from an 'upscale' club. The first girl I saw come in was bleeding from the nose, had contusions on her cheeks, and she was missing a shoe. The second girl was in worse shape. Her nipple ring had been pulled out and she was bleeding from her breast, her nose was broken, several of her false fingernails had been ripped off, and she was missing patches of hair. I was more concerned with the fact that this woman's nipple was practically ripped in half, with part of it just dangling from her boob.

"What the hell happened?" I asked. I think I was asking anyone who'd answer, instead of directing the question at a specific person.

One of the arresting officers said, "Fight."

The women were almost fully nude. We tried to get them in rooms as quickly as humanly possible because they were gathering a crowd of onlookers. We even tried to give the women blankets, but they both refused.

Although the women were in separate rooms and were guarded by officers, they somehow managed to go at each other again, after screaming through the curtains.

Right there, in the center of the corridor, these two strippers were tearing at each other and throwing punches that would have me knocked out in two seconds. The officers struggled to break them up, and finally someone paged our security team and the women were separated.

"What in the world?" asked one of the doctors, coming back from break.

"She took my money!" one of the strippers yelled.

"I was on that stage, too. It's not just your money."

"They were throwing it at me," the other countered.

"Nobody would throw money at a skank like you!"

The two tried to fight again, but one of the officers tased the woman with the loose nipple.

While the first girl was released to the officers, the second was sent upstairs for observation because she was in such bad shape. We heard a rumor that she wanted to go to surgery to fix her nipple, but her insurance said that was a cosmetic expense and they would not pay for the hospital to perform that surgery.

--B.L.
Nevada

Medicated to Work Here

I don't know how she flew under the radar for so long, but one of our pharmacists was fired, arrested, and had her license revoked because she was passing pills.

Now, she wasn't selling these stolen pills for cash or anything. And this woman never dealt to anyone outside of the hospital.

What she was doing, we all discovered, was stealing pills and trading them to coworkers in exchange of days off, PTO hours, or her preferred shifts. Accusations arose that this pharmacist had also attempted to trade narcotics and controlled substances in exchange of free cafeteria food, parking stickers, and clothing from our marketing department.

An investigation found she traded somewhere around 20 bottles of pain meds before she was caught. We're not exactly sure how she was caught, but someone told me the valet guy turned her in after she tried to bribe him to pull her car to the entrance in exchange for some Hydrocodone pills. Several of her coworkers were arrested and fired, too.

--L.D.
Georgia

I dispatched fire rescue to a caller who'd climbed a tree to help a 'stuck' cat. The cat jumped down, but the caller was then stuck 20 feet in the air.

--R.T.
Colorado

Death Threats and Percocet

I had a rough start to my day, which normally starts around five in the afternoon, but that day started around eleven in the morning. I'd gotten two hours of sleep before the school called and said my daughter was sick. She was vomiting and had a fever, so I stayed up with her and tried to nap when it looked like she was going to nap, but she ended up waking and therefore I was awake, too. My husband called and said he was going to be late from work, and the time he was to be home was time I was counting on to try to nap before my shift, which is 7p-7a.

As if being exhausted wasn't enough of a punishment for a nurse in a crazy-busy suburban ER, I stopped for a coffee on the way to work and spilled hot coffee all over my white scrubs and my cream cloth seats. I was so mad. I knew I didn't have extra scrubs at work because I kept forgetting them at the house, so I'd have to borrow the 'loaner scrubs,' which are the equivalent of being back in high school and having to wear the dingy, mismatched, ill-fitting gym clothes if you forgot yours.

By the time I pulled in the lot, it was raining, as in pouring. I didn't have an umbrella, and there were no close spots open, so I had to walk almost a block's distance from the back lot to the ER entrance. My hair was a matted mess, my makeup was a disaster, and I was cold.

As soon as I walked inside, my supervisor assigned me to a patient.

"Let me change real quick," I said.

She said there was no time, that she needed me to work on an incoming Peds code.

I was dripping water all over a coding toddler as I did chest compressions. The boy died.

After I changed my scrubs, I realized I had forgotten my badge. Here, if you forget your badge you can't do anything on your own.

You can't get to other parts of the hospital, like the supply closet or break room; you can't dispense meds, you can't even log in on some computers in our area because you have to have to scan your badge for access. On other computers, you have to enter a long number from your badge, and I still hadn't memorized mine because I was just assigned a new number, so I couldn't access half of the databases to log reports or submit orders to Central Supply. That part alone would have been enough to ruin my shift. I tried to call my husband, but he turns his phone off when he goes to bed, so that sure wasn't working.

My next patient was a male in his early thirties. He looked like a walking skeleton, thanks to years of substance abuse. He answered yes to using almost every drug I asked about, and his arms were so bruised I could hardly make out the color of his skin, though I imagine it was pasty like the rest of his skin. His eyes were sunken and he appeared malnourished. He couldn't recall the last time he'd eaten, but he refused every meal we had to offer because he specifically wanted Red Lobster. He actually told me at one point that it was my job to get him what he wanted, to which I replied nurses are not waitresses. He tried to hit me, and I then called security.

Because there was nothing medically wrong with the patient during that visit...Let me rephrase this. The patient appeared to be in a downward spiral, but he refused counseling, refused to be admitted to our rehab floor, and he refused food. He was not a model for a clean slate of health, but he presented with no ailments that would require admission during that time. Once he admitted he was seeking a Percocet script, we discharged him. He threatened to kill me, but everyone brushed it off because if I worried about every single death threat I've heard, I would be too petrified to live a normal life.

The patient left and, as it goes, more patients came and went.

That entire night was horrible. I had forgotten my lunch and was going to sneak a meal tray from the cafeteria, but the nursing supervisor started asking which patient wanted the tray, so I couldn't eat. My coworker let me use her badge so I could get to our break room, but we didn't have anything in there to eat unless I wanted to have a gourmet saltine cracker smeared with expired mustard and sriracha sauce. I must have gone through two pots of coffee on my own, which left me jittery and discombobulated. I was a freaking walking, talking mess.

    My last patient of the night was a drug overdose that came in two hours before the shift was over. Her parents, siblings, both of her boyfriends, her friends, and her classmates showed up in the ER lobby and because she was my patient, it was my job to go out there and dive in the ocean of 'I need to be back there right now because...' excuses. The woman's boyfriends ended up fighting and then some of the other people in the group became involved. Somewhere along the line, I was elbowed in the face and my front tooth chipped. I don't know if I've ever felt anything more painful than that, excluding child birth. The pain from my exposed nerve to air had me seeing stars, and because I was taken out of the game by an elbow, I couldn't get out of the way of the fighting and was knocked to the floor. I hit my head on the tile and that's the first time I've ever seriously considered quitting my job. The police were called to the lobby and the fight was broken up. I called the nursing supervisor and filed a report of my injuries, but I was not allowed to go home due to the patient load to nurse ratio. You don't hear a lot about that when you're watching these dramatized, silly medical shows, but if you're a nurse and two of your coworkers don't show up, don't expect to go home early if you have double or triple the patients you usually have, even if your arm has been chopped off. Nobody really cares about you. It's all about making sure that the really sick patients don't die and the ones who were never going to come close to dying in the first place give the hospital a positive review.

    When it was finally time to go, the nursing supervisor 'voluntold' me to stay over because someone from first shift called in. All I wanted to do was sleep. Okay, I wanted to eat and cry, too, but mainly I wanted to sleep. My husband called to tell me that my daughter was still sick and he didn't know what to do because he had to go to work. His job is strict with call ins, but after an hour of playing phone tag and both of us arguing because we were stressed, he contacted his boss and got the day off. At least that was handled.

I finally left work two hours after I was scheduled to be off. I don't know how I made it across the parking lot because I zoned out. All I knew was I went to unlock my car but realized I had never locked it in the first place. When I got in the driver's seat, I was mostly relieved that nobody had stolen my radio or gotten in my glove compartment. I had an extra stethoscope in there that ran me more than my wedding band cost, so I really was lucky that nobody hadn't stolen that.

Right as I went to place my car key in the ignition, I felt something dig into my neck and I was pinned against the seat. I instinctively pulled forward to get away, but I was choking the more I struggled. I clawed at whatever was around my neck before I caught a glimpse of a man in my rearview mirror.

The drug seeker from that night was sitting in my back seat. He was completely naked.

His clothes were on the seat next to him, wadded up in balls.

My entire life slowed. Three people passed my car and I don't know if they couldn't see that I was being strangled, or they didn't want to get involved. I knew I was going to die. I started thinking of every bad thing I'd ever done. Then I thought of meeting my husband. I thought back to our wedding. I thought of when we learned I was pregnant. I thought of my daughter's birth and her first steps and her first words and the first time she fell asleep without crying for her binkie. I thought about crying on her first day of pre-K, and I thought of all the times I'd felt frustrated because she wanted to play with me when all I wanted to do was relax on the couch and watch a movie or get through one phone conversation without her coming in the room to interrupt me. I thought about her being in the next room when the cops came to my house to tell my husband I was dead. I thought about how my little girl was going to grow up without a mother. I worried because my husband couldn't braid her hair, and he didn't know which tights to make her wear with her pink dress, and he didn't know that she had to have her pancakes cut horizontally in the mornings. I thought about my husband falling apart and packing up my belongings and how my life would somehow end up being a few boxes hidden in the attic until my daughter wanted just one more piece of me on her wedding day, a day I would miss because a drug addict was snuffing out my life.

I started hitting the steering wheel as I was blacking out. All I can remember was laying on the horn and pressing as hard as I could, while using my left hand to try to remove whatever was around my neck. After that, I remember waking up in the same trauma room the child had died in hours prior. All I could think when everyone was hovered over me was 'this is the death room.' I still thought I was going to die.

They said I was without oxygen for an estimated two minutes before someone finally came to my rescue. That person was a pregnant nurse who worked on the hospice floor. It took two minutes of hearing my horn blaring nonstop for someone to step in and help me. They rerolled the security tapes and the man who'd strangled me was on the camera when I got to work. He had been sitting in a covered bus waiting area and watched me get out of my car. We also saw that while the assault was taking place, more than ten people passed my vehicle—even when the horn was sounding. Only one person stopped to help. Thankfully, she thought quickly and used her car key to stab the man in the arm until he released the shoe string he was using to strangle me.

I was offered workman's comp, a week off from work, and was instructed to attend mandatory counseling. I quit my job and now work in a doctor's office. The patient who almost took my life escaped from the scene that day. He was arrested a few weeks later when he came back to the ER and someone recognized him. He told the cops that he 'maybe could have' tried to kill me, but he couldn't remember because of all the cocaine he'd recently used. He was sent to a rehab center, and after I saw he was released, I stopped following his case or trying to figure out what happened to him. Justice was not served in my case, but at least I have my life.

I will forever be indebted to the brave woman who risked her own life so that I could have mine.

--K.W.
New York

Push!

I love nurses, and that's the God's honest truth. There are times, however, that I meet nurses whom I do not believe should be in the healthcare profession. One such example of this was a woman fresh out of college. She had been working on the OB floor approximately three weeks at the time of this recollection.

At 3:05 A.M., I received three consecutive pages and missed two calls to my cell phone. It was not that I am an inattentive sleeper, but that the calls and pages were within a three-minute span. This generally does not occur unless one of my patients is in distress or has been involved in an accident. Because of this, I began dressing myself as I phoned the hospital.

The answering nurse was panting and could not seem to catch her breath. I instructed her to calm herself and we practiced a few deep breaths together until she could gather composure.

"Tell me what the situation is," I said.

"Ms. Smith is here, and she says she has to push right now. I'd say she's dilated to an eight right now. We need you to come in as fast as you can."

"How long has she been admitted?" I questioned.

"About an hour."

I rushed across town, eager to deliver Ms. Smith's child. It was pertinent that I was there for her. I generally do not become personally involved in my patients' lives, but Ms. Smith was a tragic case. Her husband recently passed, and her pregnancy and overall health suffered greatly from the loss of her spouse. She did not have family, nor did her late husband. While Ms. Smith did have friends, she confided in me that she felt alone and was scared. I promised I would help her through her birth and assured her she was strong and capable of bringing this child into the world.

The nurse who had paged me met me in the hall as soon as I stepped out of the elevator.

"She's struggling," said the nurse.

I cleaned up and gloved up before entering the room. Ms. Smith's legs were already in stirrups and she was straining. Her breathing was erratic and a CNA was rubbing an ice cube across the patient's forehead, while coaching her on steady breathing.

Ms. Smith cried when she saw me. "I can't do this," she said.

I nodded as I crossed the room and assured her that she very well could and would.

"Let's take a look," I said.

When I took a seat on the stool at the foot of the bed, I glanced once at Ms. Smith's privates and immediately shot a stone-cold glare to the nurse who'd called me.

"You're kidding me," I said.

"I told you," replied the nurse. "She's dilated and said she needs to push. She wanted you here for the delivery."

I shook my head. "You woke me up at three in the morning for this?"

Ms. Smith immediately began sobbing. "You promised you would be here."

"For the birth," I replied laughingly, trying to ease her discomfort, "which is still some time away."

"But she said she had to push," the nurse argued. "And she's dilated."

"I can't feel anything but pressure," Ms. Smith stated. "What's happening? Do you see anything? Do you see the baby?"

"Ms. Smith, I'm not exactly sure how this mistake occurred," I said, glancing at the nurse, "but that pressure you feel is a bowel movement."

With assistance, the patient excreted a rather large bowel movement. She did state that she had been constipated, and we could see why.

Long story short here: the nurse called me because she was looking at the 'wrong hole,' may we say for the sake of 'safe for work.' She did not remain on at the facility for much longer, but I am unsure if she left on her own accord or was terminated. Ms. Smith gave birth to a healthy baby a few more than twenty hours later.

--W.B.
New Mexico

Deluxe

After a long night of chasing idiots who decided to make me work to arrest them, I went through the drive through of a local taco place. I ordered two deluxe chicken tacos. These tacos are the best in town, and I was craving them all night.

Now, on this place's menu, a deluxe chicken taco is listed as the following: premium chicken marinated in savory spices, grilled to perfection, placed on a toasted hand-ground corn tortilla, and topped with delicious avocado slices, roasted tomatoes, creamy chipotle sauce, and a three-cheese blend.

When I pulled to the window, the clerk inside took one look at me, laughed, and said, "You sure you're the one with the deluxe tacos?"

I nodded. "I've been waiting all day for my fix."

The guy laughed excitedly, nodded in return, and said, "Cool. Cool."

I moved to pay him, but he shook his head and said, "It's already been handled. Nobody told you that?"

I didn't think much of it, really, because from time to time, we all get free or discounted food and/or services. I never expect free services from anyone, but I'd be lying if I said that I wasn't extremely appreciative of the gesture from the people in our community.

It took me about a block to realize that I couldn't smell the tacos from the white paper bag resting in the passenger seat. I started thinking of the short conversation I had with the clerk. As soon as I pulled up to the station, I opened the bag to not find tacos, but to find it halfway full of blue envelopes. Inside those blue envelopes were small bags filled with heroin. In total, there were 116 envelopes. In hindsight, maybe it wasn't such a great idea to tell him I had needed my fix, huh?

Of course, I went back to the taco joint to complain that my order had been mixed up with another customer's. When the clerk confessed that he thought I was the 'pickup dude,' we waited until the real 'pickup dude' drove up and we hauled him in, too.

--V.A.
Illinois

Possession

I am a devote Christian. My father was a pastor, and I have a near-immaculate track record of sermon attendance, which stems back to my childhood. My apologies if this sounds like boastful pride; I am merely wishing to add this because I feel it adds to why I felt so terrorized by the story I have sent to you.

Mr. Smith was transferred to our ICU following a rather incredible ER experience. He was allegedly discovered nude, running through the streets, and he was hit by a truck. He sustained a massive amount of injuries, from internal bleeding to broken bones. Mr. Smith sustained life-threatening head trauma.

What was incredible about all of this is that Mr. Smith was somewhat lucid during his ER visit, at least at first. He repeatedly begged ER staff not to let 'him' take him, that he wasn't ready. He apologized for 'being weak.'

Mr. Smith then slipped away and was placed on life support. The very few members of his family were informed that Mr. Smith was in a permanent vegetative state. He would never recover. Though we all like to believe miracles are possible, and though I fully believe in the power of my God, we sometimes must look at the scientific data to see that we can't hold on to the less than one-percent chance of limited recovery.

This patient's family, understandably, had difficulty reaching a decision regarding his life plan. They asked for one week. If they did not see progress, they agreed to terminate Mr. Smith's life support and allow him to pass.

For five nights, Mr. Smith was motionless. Machines breathed for him. He was hooked to countless monitors. We continued our rounds and checked vitals just the same.

On the sixth night, I entered Mr. Smith's room and noticed something on the floor beside his bed. Upon closer inspection, I realized it was simply a piece of scrap paper one of the other nurses had dropped. I shoved it in my pocket and stood from my kneeling position. As I turned, I screamed.

Mr. Smith was sitting upright in his bed, only it wasn't Mr. Smith. I have thought this through at least a dozen times, and despite never having met this man before, I could tell you this was not who he once was. His eyes were dark and there was a certain…I don't know how else to say it. This man looked evil. It was as if evil seeped from his every pore as he was sitting there. He had a creepy smirk on his face, like he was taunting me. I think it was, whatever was in him.

Immediately, I started reciting the Lord's Prayer, and I felt stuck. Every part of me wanted to move, but I didn't feel like I could. I don't mean physically, because I think I could have run from the room, but mentally, I could not tell my legs to move.

"You dumb c**ts need to just let him die," Mr. Smith said. "Let him die, and let me have him."

The man laughed, and I closed my eyes tightly. When I opened them, Mr. Smith was in a lying position again.

I notified my supervisor of this and she called the nursing supervisor. He then called mental health because he thought I was having a psychotic break.

While I was telling my story for a third time to the mental health counselor, Mr. Smith passed away. When he died, the power to his room went out. Technicians went in and out of that room for three days and found nothing wrong with the wiring. Nothing in the room would work, not the monitors, not the outlets, and not even the battery-powered BP monitor or clocks. The power turned on in the middle of the third night, seemingly on its own.

I was instructed never to talk about this to Mr. Smith's family or anyone outside of the hospital. I was scared to death of mentioning it, anyway, just as much as I was afraid of meeting what I've since interpreted as the devil.

Another nurse on the floor visited my home unexpectedly about a month after this happened. She told me she didn't want to say anything at work because she didn't think anyone would believe her, but she said that while she was in Mr. Smith's room to check his vitals and change his catheter, she heard whispers that called her name and told her to 'unplug him.' She said that she turned toward Mr. Smith just as she was leaving the room and swore the man smiled and winked at her.

--Initials and location withheld at request

My critical patient's wife left the ER so that she could go buy the set of dishes she'd been eyeing, now that it was Black Friday. We stabilized the patient and flew him out while his wife was gone shopping.

--L.R.
New York

Unbelievable

The strangest arrest I've ever made happened when a cocaine dealer called 911. He reported parents had given their eight-year-old money to buy them drugs under the threat that they would kill him if he returned empty-handed. When the dealer refused to do business with the child, the kid began sobbing and pleading with the dealer.

This dealer told me that he had 'moral obligations' and refused to do business with children. He said he felt so bad for the kid that he knew he had to do something. The D.A. cut a deal with the man, and the child was taken out of his home by child services. His parents were also arrested.

--T.F.
Florida

In the middle of a tubal ligation (with complications), our surgeon put down his utensils and said, "You know what? I quit."

I didn't know what to do. The nursing supervisor had to stat page another surgeon in to assess and finish the surgery.

The surgeon faced charges for endangering the patient and was in a lawsuit with both the patient and the hospital.

--N.M.
California

Duck, Duck, Goose

In the ER one night, one of our patients became disruptive. We don't have security at our facility, so we threatened to call the police. The patient promised to calm down, but that didn't last too long.

As I was ordering crutches for another patient, some of the nurses started screaming from the other side of the room. I turned my head to see my patient running behind staff and other patients.

He screamed, "Wedgie!" before effectively performing said action (pulling a person's pants and/or underpants upward from behind).

This patient continued around the emergency room giving people wedgies. Nobody could catch him. The ER looked like a preschool game of 'Duck, Duck, Goose,' with nurses, doctors, and patients' family members chasing after this guy.

At one point, the patient picked up a pair of scissors from a crash cart and grabbed one of our nurses. He threatened to slit her throat if we refused to discharge him. Instead, he snatched a chunk of her hair and cut it off next to her scalp. This would be sad to see on any woman, but the woman in question had hair down to her mid-section, and she had to basically shave her head to start all over again because the man butchered her hair.

The police arrived and shot a bean bag at the patient. He was restrained and transferred for an involuntary psychiatric hold at a larger, more equipped facility.

--X.A.
Alabama

First World Slum Hospital

When I moved to the West Coast, I knew I wanted to continue my nursing career, so I applied at several hospitals within a popular city in California. I received call backs from every hospital to which I applied but would not decide until I toured the facility, at least the general vicinity in which I would be working.

The first hospital I visited was nothing short of a night terror. I was supposed to meet a member of HR in the evening, which I found to be a remarkably odd meeting time. When I arrived to the hospital, I was informed the HR member 'changed her mind' and a nurse handed me a badge with another nurse's name on it and told me to feel free to walk around and visit other floors. These people obviously entrusted me with someone's personal badge and with visiting areas otherwise restricted to the general public without proper clearance.

From the get-go, I could tell this place was not in tip-top shape, but the facility was older and I thought perhaps they could not receive funding for renovations, or thought perhaps they asked for funding for medical necessities instead. I noted holes in the walls, missing chunks of wallpaper you'd expect to see in your great-grandmother's bedroom, cigarette butts along the hall floors, and even saw blood smeared in several places (on signs, walls, and furniture) as I made my way to the emergency room, where I would be an overnight RN.

Few patients were in the waiting room as I passed it. The clerks at the registration desk were arguing with a gentleman who, in my professional opinion, needed immediate intervention. He had cut his fingers to the point that one was hanging on by tendons and the others were mangled. Registration handed the man a clipboard and dryly instructed him to fill out the paperwork and then they would 'see' about getting him a nurse.

I introduced myself to the registration clerks and asked if the ER was at full capacity in the back, to which one woman replied, "No, but he's going to wait because I said he's going to wait."

She couldn't care less about the patient, and that alone should have been enough to send me packing. I suppose I held out in hopes that the hospital's care providers would show more compassion and sense of urgency, but they showed far less than what I viewed at the registration desk.

In back, elderly patients, unable to walk unassisted, were struggling to walk to the restroom. Some of the nurses were reading, while some were playing on their phones. One nurse was standing in the doorway of a treatment room and said, "If you don't like it, get your stuff and get out. I said the emesis bags are in the supply closet, and I don't feel like going to get more. Puke in the trash can or leave. Stop wasting my time."

I was appalled.

Patients were moaning and crying out from every direction. I heard an elderly patient crying and calling out that she had been lying in her own excrement for two hours and nobody would help her.

There was no doctor in sight. When I asked a nurse if the doctor was with a patient, she laughed and said, "Honey, the doctor left two hours ago. We're without one until the next guy comes in, if he decides to come in on time."

I asked if the doctor on shift quit, to which she laughed again and said, "No. He went to play golf and get dinner. We all kind of leave whenever we feel like it. It's really a nice setup we have going for us."

The emergency room was left without a doctor, can you believe it? What if a trauma or code arrived? What if someone needed treatment that only a doctor could provide? These nurses were left on their own to provide care they were not able to legally provide at other hospitals—any hospital, to my knowledge. Would these patients truly be left to die? It sure seemed that way.

I witnessed another nurse speaking to a patient. She kept calling the patient Joan Smitty. The patient corrected the nurse by explaining her name was Jane Smith, not Joan

Smitty. The nurse told, "I'll call you what I want to call you. Now get moving, or you're not being seen."

As I continued around the ER, I saw roaches and a rat scurried across the hall and disappeared behind a cabinet. I was not put off as much regarding the pests as I was the blatant acceptance of them in the workplace. Nobody made a comment like, 'We should notify someone,' or, 'It looks like someone needs to spray again.' Nobody cared.

My last straw at this hospital was when I went upstairs and somehow ended up on the OB floor. A father was screaming at a nurse after I watched the nurse hand a newborn to the wrong mother in the wrong room. She only went back for the child after the dad rightfully threw a fit and told the nurse that was *his* child, not the other patient's child. She hadn't bothered to check the identification bands and didn't seem to care at all about her mistake.

I took a position at a well-known hospital there in the city and love my job. I bounce between the ER and OB, and I've never been happier in a career. As for the first hospital I toured, I hope the place is shut down sooner than later.

--E.T.
California

The strangest call I've ever received was regarding a naked man push-mowing someone's front lawn at three in the morning.

The nude perpetrator was arrested for public intox.

--D.B.
Delaware

__Miracle of Life__

If your audience cannot understand the importance of the need for more funding and resources for mental health, my experience will hopefully allow them to.

Jane visited our ER on a regular basis. She was diagnosed with schizophrenia and regularly presented with hallucinations (seen and heard), regularly participated in self-harming, and she always begged for help. The problem was, we are an inner-city facility and no matter how hard we tried, we could not keep Jane for more than a day or two at a time, and we could not find a facility that would take her in. She was in desperate need of assistance, but we couldn't help her. She couldn't afford medication, she jumped from residence to residence, and she coped with her illness by participating in illegal drugs, which she said helped her calm the voices in her head, but did not assist her with lashing out violently or visual hallucinations.

We knew it was a problem when Jane tested positive for pregnancy. Several of us spent hours and weeks calling to facilities in the area and even out of state, but Jane did not have insurance, and with her drug usage and now pregnancy, nobody could offer her the residence she needed. She was essentially on her own. At the time of her pregnancy discovery, Jane stated she was living with her boyfriend. She casually told us of how he hit and kicked her, put cigarettes out on her arms and legs…but she denied this was abuse. She stated that was her boyfriend's 'love language.'

Jane was arrested a month or two later because she stabbed her boyfriend. The system failed her and released her because there was no place for her to go, with facilities citing her violent behavior, drug usage, and pregnancy as factors of denial. Jane was left to the streets, and someone told me Jane had been living in a condemned building because she had nowhere else to go.

When Jane was around 22 weeks pregnant, she visited the ER and threatened to harm herself. We could not accept her as a patient to our mental health unit because that floor was full. The nursing supervisor did not feel comfortable admitting Jane to another floor because she needed extra security precautions—for herself and for our staff. Unfortunately, we had to turn Jane away. We gave her a card for a nearby women's shelter and told her to seek help.

Jane returned a few hours later. We received word from incoming patients that Jane was standing in our parking lot with a weapon. When security arrived, they called 911. Jane was holding a gun to her head.

Despite first responders' attempts to disarm Jane, she pulled the trigger and committed suicide just a few steps from the emergency room entrance. One of our doctors was concerned for Jane's fetus and demanded that her body be brought inside.

The doctor rapidly cut into Jane's abdomen and performed a crude version of an emergency C-section on the deceased woman. Her child was placed in NICU but was thriving well and was then placed in the care of Child Services.

I think of Jane daily and at times multiple times per day. All of this could have been avoided. Some have stated their beliefs that Jane's child is 'better off' in the care of Child Services, but I can't help to think that maybe Jane's child would have been able to grow up with her own mother if assistance had been available to treat her mother's illness.

--K.C.
New Jersey

(Hot) Broken Water

A handful of readers sent in stories regarding outrageous things men and/or family members have done or said while that special lady was in labor. Here they are:

- We had to call security to remove our patient's sister from the room because she and the patient got in a fist fight when the patient announced what she planned to name her child. Apparently, the name she picked for her child was the name her pregnant sister picked out for her (the sister) own child, who was due just a few weeks later. (L.T., North Carolina)

- A new mother broke down in tears because she had told her husband to throw some underwear in the 'go' bag before they left for the hospital. He packed three thongs. We gave the new mom a comfy pair of granny panties. (Z.R., Indiana)

- One mother threw a book at her husband when he complained that labor was 'taking forever' and he was 'exhausted.' Dad had to go down to the ER for three stitches to the face. (P.Y., Ohio)

- I went to the room to give the patient ice chips. Her boyfriend followed me to the hall and asked me if I wanted to go out sometime. His girlfriend gave birth two hours later. He asked me again before mom and baby were discharged. Ew. (K.T., Arizona)

- The patient's husband showed up with the girlfriend he'd picked up while his wife was six months pregnant and demanded she sign the divorce papers. It was a nightmare. We had to call the police to make him and the girlfriend leave. (R.B., Washington)

- My patient's husband took one of her pillows while she was getting the epidural and caused the needle to slip during the injection. We were able to successfully administer the epidural, but his wife was (understandably) irate. Dad slept through his baby's birth. (G.L., Georgia)

- The patient's boyfriend yelled at her while she was loudly working through a contraction because he couldn't hear what his bookie was saying over the phone. (K.P., Utah)

- My patient was dehydrated from vomiting for six hours straight, when her husband asked if she could 'try not to push' while he went out for lunch. (W.B., Illinois)

- Patient's family brought booze to the waiting room, got drunk, and the patient's husband passed out and broke the waiting room table. We called the cops and the patient was crying because nobody was sober and nobody was in the room with her when she gave birth. (J.O., South Carolina)

- When the baby emerged, the patient's husband became woozy and asked, "What's all over him? Why isn't he clean, like on TV?" He fainted and we spent more time tending to him than talking to his wife about her newborn. (R.M., North Dakota)

- The patient's mother pulled me aside and asked, "Would it be too late for an abortion? She really wanted to wait until she was 30 to have kids." I replied, "Uh, 39 weeks and eight centimeters dilated is too late, yes." I walked away to keep from smacking her. (F.C., Alabama)

- One husband told his wife to 'stop complaining and making [labor] a bigger deal than it [was].' He said his cattle give birth all the time and don't make nearly as much 'racket' as his wife was making. She told him in not-so-nice words that maybe he should go sleep with his cattle, then. He shut up. (T.R., Iowa)

__Paging Doctor...Oh__

Where I work, everyone around here humps like they're trying to repopulate a broken world, I swear. There's always drama because so-and-so is sleeping with so-and-so, who so-and-so thought was being faithful and only wanted him/her. HR has become involved with relationships so many times that you'd think they'd separate us by genders, but obviously, they can't do that, so nothing they do is really going to make everyone stop sleeping around.

One night, our ER was flirting (again) with a float from Surgical. We all figured they'd already done the dirty, but rumor got out that they had only been flirting heavily and hadn't gone all the way. I'm not sure what stopped them. Someone suggested it was that the doctor was married and had three kids, but it had never stopped him from having a side piece before. The girl from Surgical seemed religious, always quoting Bible passages and stuff, so I thought maybe she was saving herself.

Our department was dead at one point. We cleaned up our station and scrubbed down beds, stocked the crash carts, just made sure everything was taken care of, and then we relaxed. Someone brought down a projector from the meeting room and rigged their laptop to it, so we streamed *The Hunger Games* on the far wall. Someone else made popcorn, and we 'borrowed' a few sodas from the patient fridge.

Probably about half through the movie, as it usually goes, we got busy. At first, we didn't think too much of the doctor being gone. We thought he'd gone to take his break or maybe went to the restroom. After fifteen minutes, we paged him for a child experiencing labored breathing, but he never answered.

We started to get worried, so someone paged the nursing supervisor, and she sent out a house wide page to form a 'search party' to find the doctor. I guess she thought he could have been injured or taken hostage or something.

While the nursing supervisor was on the phone, calling the head of the hospital, the ceiling rattled above a section of hallway that had been taped off. The floor above us experienced a water main burst, and the ceiling was thought to be weakened.

Now, you'd think that knowing that would be enough to tell you not to, oh I don't know, sneak in that area and have sex with the girl from Surgical on the water-damaged floor, but apparently some people don't have much sense. The doctor and the girl from Surgical fell through the ceiling and landed on the ER floor. The doctor wasn't wearing pants, and the girl from Surgical was completely nude, except for the ankle-high socks she was wearing.

Both had to be registered as patients, and the girl from Surgical had to get sutures on several places of her body because she scraped metal framing when she fell. Our doctor shattered his knee in the fall.

The hospital couldn't afford to lose the doctor, nor could they afford the lawsuit the girl from Surgical threatened if she was fired and the doctor wasn't, so both were written up and ordered to attend a mandatory seminar on the importance of refraining from sexual harassment and relationships in the workplace.

As far as I know, the doctor's wife never found out about her husband's escapades. He told her he fell down the stairs.

--S.C.
Nebraska

To Avoid Arrest

Dispatch received a call from an LEO requesting immediate medical transport. He was performing a traffic stop when he noticed the subject had been acting suspiciously, i.e. jittery, laughing nervously, all-around behaving as if he was guilty of something more than speeding. When the officer requested the man step out of the vehicle and allow a canine unit to perform a drug search, the man complied. While the officer was retrieving his canine partner, the subject ingested approximately 10 grams of methamphetamines.

When my partner and I arrived on scene, just off the highway, the subject was on the ground, convulsing. He was continually vomiting and despite being rolled to his side, he was aspirating his vomit.

The patient died during transport.

To this day, I still wonder if the patient believed he would live through that. In his mind, I suppose ingesting the drugs seemed like a way to avoid arrest.

-- Initials and location withheld at request

A woman arrived at the ER at three in the morning because she stated she took eleven home pregnancy tests, all of which were positive. This was an 'emergency' because she did not want to be pregnant. She wanted us to test so that we could conclude the eleven home tests were false positives.

They weren't, of course. She was with child.

--D.H.
Oregon

Mother and Wife of the Year

The Smith family frequently visited the ER for abdominal pain. At times, Mr. Smith and his two children would present with vomiting as well. Mrs. Smith refused to allow nursing staff to fetch her family water or blankets. She insisted on doting on her family while they were ill.

After a few months of coming in once a month for abdominal pain and/or vomiting, the Smith family began frequenting the ER a few times per week. Mrs. Smith appeared frazzled, with dark circles under her eyes from lack of sleep. Gray hairs started popping up on her head. She was getting deep wrinkles around her eyes.

Fed up of scans and blood tests showing no signs of illness, the doctor on call ordered a full blood panel on Mr. Smith and his ill children. In Lab, the three were asked about their eating habits. Dad said the family always became sick after the mother cooked or prepared their takeout dinners.

After Mr. Smith's 16th visit to the ER, he returned on the 17th visit without Mrs. Smith or their children—and he brought a slice of pecan pie his wife had baked for the family. He requested a test of the pie, and Lab sent the food off to another lab at a steep price.

It paid off.

Mrs. Smith had been lacing her family's suppers with pesticide. She was arrested and admitted that she thought she could poison her family, increasing the dosage over time, until they were 'gone.' She did this because she was 'sick and tired of taking care of them.'

--J.I.
New Jersey

My partner was fired because we responded at 02:30 to a 30-something-year-old patient who said she couldn't sleep. When she repeated her 'problem' to my partner, he said, "That's so weird. I can't sleep, either, because idiots like you keep calling 911 instead of taking some freakin' Unisom."

He went down a legend at the station and with the ER.

--Initials and location withheld at request

Ouchie

We received a suicide attempt one evening. The twenty-something female slit her wrists with a razor blade, but her attempt to take her own life was thwarted when her roommate unexpectedly came home and found her.

The patient was a banshee in the ER. She screamed and squirmed so much when we tried to insert the IV that we had to restrain her. This was difficult because we had to attach the four-point restraints on her forearms rather than her wrists.

When the doctor stuck the patient with a numbing injection, she spat on him.

She said she was going to sue the hospital because we were hurting her with needles. Apparently, the patient could handle taking a razor blade to herself, but she couldn't handle injections or needle sticks because 'they hurt,' and she didn't think we were being 'fair' to her by subjecting her to that sort of pain.

I still can't wrap my head around that.

--A.D.
Location withheld at request

Oopsie

I work at a 24-hour pharmacy and generally man the midnight to eight A.M. shift. I've noticed this is the prime-time for narco seekers to come in. Every now and then, I'll see a mom come in with a prescription for her sick kid, but mostly, it's the same people over and over, the ones with slips from different hospitals all over the county, all for pain meds.

This one night, a guy came to the counter with a prescription. He looked like he was in bad shape. He handed me a slip of paper with a bunch of scribbles. It was from the local hospital. He was impatient as I filled his prescription. He tapped on the window at least four times, and I told him it would be a few minutes because I had another order to fill, and then I had to count out his pills and put the order in the system.

When I finally gave the man his prescription, he opened the bottle and poured pills from the bottle into his mouth. He swallowed some and coughed up the rest, sending pink capsules flying all over the carpet and counter.

"What is this?" he yelled. "Is this some kind of joke?"

I wasn't following and told him that.

"I wanted pain pills," he said.

"The prescription was for allergy medicine," I explained. "That's what I gave you."

He argued. "No, I wrote Benadryl. That's what they gave my sister when she broke her leg. If I wanted this crap, I would've wrote that instead."

"Benadryl is an allergy medicine," I said.

"I want the white pills. The ones for pain," he said. "That's what I wrote. That's what I want."

This idiot busted himself. What made him dumber was that I told him it was my mistake, and I asked him to have a seat while I went back to correct his order. I called the police and he was arrested for stealing a prescription pad from the ER, where they had denied him Hydrocodone.

   --U.L.
Utah

We've Got Cows

In the late-90s, I was dispatched to assess and transport a male with head trauma. It was unclear at the time of dispatch what caused the trauma. When I arrived on scene, it wasn't much clearer, let me just tell you that. I guess it was clear what did the damage, just not clear how it occurred.

On scene, which was in the middle of a pasture, the guy's grown children were surrounding him and one was holding a tee shirt to a gaping wound on the top of his balding head. Two of his daughters were crying, and the third adult child-a son-stood kept kicking at a crumpled metal sign that lay next to bleeding dad.

"What happened?" I asked. The second I turned off the paved road a few minutes earlier, I expected to see a terrible farm accident. We're in farm country, and we must get at least a half dozen fatal calls every spring to summer. It's worse during harvesting.

The son shrugged. "Dunno. Jane looked out the window at just the right time and saw him fall down. We haven't been able to bring him to."

Jane released her left hand from the tee shirt on dad's head to point at the sign. "That thing fell from the sky."

Jane's sister tearfully asked, "Think it could've come from an airline?"

I glanced at the sign as my partner was trudging through the pasture. It sure didn't seem like any sign I'd ever imagine on a flight. It was a distressed metal sign that had a picture of a cherry pie on the front and it said '$2 per slice.'

"Not unless you know an airline that serves pie in flight," I said, with the shake of my head.

"Need ammonia caps," I called to my partner.

She waved a packet of ammonia inhalant in the air. I could always count on her. If she was ever behind, she was always arriving just as I was realizing what the patient needed.

We brought John to and explained that we were going to transport him to the emergency room. He refused to go to county because he said his sister-in-law worked there and he hated her, which we took as a sign that he was not in critical condition. John was losing a significant amount of blood and was woozy. He told us the same story, about how he was out in the pasture calling for his dogs, when a sign 'done fell out of nowhere' and sliced his head open.

John received 11 staples to close his wound.

What I found remarkable about this whole thing is that someone from town recognized that sign from a few towns over. That sign used to hang in a restaurant, before a tornado destroyed it a few days earlier. John's family went to see someone at the university and he said it was completely possible that though the weather had appeared calm in our neck of the woods, that the sky was still carrying debris from the storm. It was just John's great bout of bad luck that brought the sign to whack him on the noggin in broad daylight.

--P.G.
Nebraska

Back in the late-80s, early-90s, we had a guy try to pay his traffic ticket with a bag of drugs. Mind you, he came to court to try to get out of the ticket, and when he couldn't, he tried to offer the *judge* the drugs as payments.

I was the judge.

--G.A.

Location withheld at request

Get it, Granny

My partner and I (both females) transported a female in her late 90s to the local ER because her SNF (Skilled Nursing Facility) called in a report of Alt Loc (Altered Level of Consciousness) following a fall that had gone unreported for four hours. Per the nursing facility, they stated they would not have to report the fall because they could 'handle' the patient…Well, until she started acting the way she was. The patient warranted a call to 911 after she was found gyrating on men in the activities room.

This patient was a firecracker. The entire way to the hospital, she chattered on about 'sexy men' and told us about her past sexual conquests, along with those she 'stupidly' missed the chance to have. By the time we reached the ER, my partner and I were crying from how hilarious this woman was.

When we reached the hospital, the patient was more lively than ever. She was groping techs by the rear ends and she even grabbed at her doctor's penis!

She said, "Come on, baby, show me what you got."

The nurses were trying to keep straight faces as the doctor blushed, but none of us could stop laughing, even though it was obviously a serious situation that a conservative old woman would behave in such manner.

We had to go on another run, but when we checked back with the ER later, we learned the patient was diagnosed with a UTI and that, in part with the fall, was thought to have caused her altered behavior. She had a note on her door that said female staff only, due to her handsy tendencies.

--M.W.
West Virginia

As I was performing the ultrasound to confirm my patient's pregnancy, she turned to her boyfriend and asked, "How much do you think someone would pay us for it?"

They continued to have a discussion about selling the baby to the 'highest bidder.'

The patient went into preterm labor due to her drug usage and the baby was born an addict, but the child was adopted by a loving couple.

--J.S.
Florida

Wow AND Ow

We received a patient who called 911 but passed out before he could explain what had happened. Medics told us they found lye next to the patient. When we received the young patient, we figured the burns would be to his hands or facial region, due to either mixing without using gloves or experiencing backsplash.

I was not at all prepared to see that the patient's genitals were essentially mutilated. By the time we removed his clothes to see what we were dealing with, the patient's penis looked like a hot dog that had been left on the grill for too long. His testicles and inner thighs were not in much better condition.

"What the hell?" asked our doctor, upon entering the room.

We didn't know. The paramedics didn't know. We started thinking the patient could have experienced body dysmorphia or something, a condition that left him feeling unsatisfied with his body. Maybe he was trying to castrate himself? We didn't know. We simply had no idea and weren't sure what to do next.

The doctor ordered us to don our PPE gear and then attempt to clean the chemical from the patient's extremities. We thought it was best to let the patient remain unconscious during this procedure. His vitals were decent, but he was indeed in shock.

It wasn't as simple as brushing crushed lye from the patient's penis. The chemical was mixed with blood, which further burned him. As we moved closer, we could detect an odor that a tech identified as drain cleaner.

"What was this poor boy doing?" one of us asked.

We filled a bottle with cool water and irrigated the site. This is when the patient came to and began screaming bloody murder. His heart rate shot up and his blood pressure was through the roof. A blood vessel in the patient's eye burst.

"Put him out," the doctor ordered.

As we were gathering sedating meds, the doctor asked the patient what happened.

"You have to tell us," the doctor said. "We need to know what you were doing and what you mixed."

The patient stated he mixed lye and drain cleaner because his girlfriend was diagnosed with genital herpes, and he thought he could get rid of the herpes by 'cleaning' them off. He did not realize the lye and drain cleaner mixture would burn his skin. When it started hurting, he said he dialed 911 and stated he needed assistance, but he couldn't finish telling the dispatcher what was wrong because, "It really, really hurt. Like, it hurt bad."

There was no saving the man's penis. The chemicals had burned through two layers of skin and he contracted an infection while in ICU. Last I knew, he was slated for reconstructive surgery.

What's worse about all of this is that most everyone in the medical field is aware that you can't 'wash' Herpes away. I feel so bad for that young man because he honestly didn't have an idea that what he was doing was a stupid idea that wouldn't work, anyway.

-- Initials and location withheld at request

Real dispatch:

Puppy stuck under couch.

--W.V.C.
Ohio

One More Time

We received word of an incoming OD. She was administered Narcan during transport. When she arrived in our ER, she was alert, but we wanted to tape her mouth shut.

This patient was angry that medics 'ruined her party,' simply because they ruined her high. She continued screaming threats that we all 'owed' her for the money she 'wasted' on her heroin.

What was interesting about this patient was that we had seen her a week prior. She stated she wanted to get clean, but planned shooting up 'one more time.'

We were in the process of calling the police when a CNA entered the room and shouted for help.

When we rushed to the room, the patient was seizing and foaming from the mouth.

The second batch of heroin she ingested had been laced with Fentanyl. We did all we could to save the patient, but the outcome was not in our hands. The patient expired within minutes of ingesting the drug.

--N.C.
Virginia

Arachnophobia

A man carried in a febrile woman one morning, and I could smell the wound on her leg before I could see it. The woman was sure she was bitten by a brown recluse, but this wound did not look like any recluse bite I had ever seen. Our doctor took a look at the woman's oozing, cracked, and necrotic wound and said it was indeed possible it was the result of a recluse bite left untreated.

The patient's fiancé stated they could not afford professional medical treatment, so they consulted homeopathic remedies online. Home treatment included smothering the wound with lard, oils, and spices. After three and a half weeks, the patient sprung a fever that went over 105-degrees, and her fiancé insisted upon visiting the ER.

Our patient started babbling about her upcoming wedding, that was to take place in four days. She had ordered a traditional

Filipino wedding gown that was shipped from the Phillipines. We later discovered the spider responsible for her wound shipped with the dress. Her fiancé found it when he went home to pack some of the patient's belongings for her hospital admission. He brought it to the ER with him, and our doctor asked one of his friends from university to identify the species.

Unfortunately, due to the length of time the wound was left untreated, the patient's leg had to be amputated, and she postponed her wedding. She was distraught that attempting to follow her culture's tradition resulted in her life changing so drastically.

-- Initials and location withheld at request

The Devil

I had to go to our morgue. Our morgue is basically our whole basement, locked at the top of the stairs, and the elevator down is also locked by a number pad.

When I got downstairs, I couldn't remember where the light switches were, so I blindly felt along the wall and stumbled into exam tables and roll carts.

I thought I found the switch to flip on some overhead lights, but I accidentally turned on a UV light affixed to one of the exam tables. The room was still almost completely pitch black.

In the corner of the room, I spotted beady little devil eyes staring straight at me, and I screamed like a little girl. I am a 6'2" tall male and weigh 300 pounds.

The eyes moved toward me and I got it in my head that there was a demon down in the morgue. I tried to run back to the elevator, but I tripped over something, fell, and knocked myself out.

When my coworkers came looking for me, they found me unconscious on the floor.

The 'devil' eyes belonged to a cat. We're still not sure how the stray got down to the morgue.

I have since refused to go to the morgue at night. Another orderly will have to do that because that's a big 'no' from me.

--T.S.
Texas

Like the story about the Icy Hot guy, we had a patient learn not to use Vicks Rub as lubricant. She cried for hours.

--D.A.
Wyoming

Unlicensed Driver

We frequently receive ETOH drivers on New Year's Eve, whether they are transported to us via EMS or the police. I've seen a 92-year-old drunk driver, and it was common to receive patients in their teens.

What was uncommon was the 10-year-old boy who was transported for ETOH and driving.

While his parents were at the bar, ringing in a new year, the 10-year-old was left alone in his duplex. Bored and angry that his parents refused to allow his friends to stay the night or allow him to stay the night with his friends, he helped himself to his father's whisky and then borrowed his mother's minivan.

The pre-teen crashed the van three blocks from his house and caused a fire hydrant to flush. He just so happened to wreck across the street from a police officer's house, and the officer held the boy until EMS could arrive. The boy's BAC was almost double the legal limit for an adult.

The child did not appear to have difficulty ridding the alcohol from his system, as he vomited uncontrollably for an hour before falling asleep.

I don't know what happened to the child, but I know his parents were arrested for leaving him alone and not locking up their alcohol.

--Initials and location withheld at request

Coke Head

My first patient of the night was this guy who lined up unopened soda cans against a tree and tried to make them explode by shooting rocks from a slingshot at them.

The guy hit a can with a rock, which sent the can flying into the tree. I guess the can hit a rusty nail protruding from the tree and poked a hole in it. With the carbonation and pressure, the can flew across the yard and hit the guy in the face.

He was a little bruised up and one of his teeth were loose, but he lived.

Dumbest person I've ever met.

--J.C.
South Dakota

Throwing shotgun shells in a bonfire is NOT a good idea.

GSWs to three bystanders, including a critical injury.

I'm pretty sure these adults learned their lesson.

--A.M.
Kentucky

WHY?

I was the doctor on shift when a sobbing mother brought in her six-week-old daughter. The newborn was bleeding from both lobes. Blood was running down the mother's bare arms.

I will never understand why the mother did this, but she pierced her baby's ears and placed silver hoops. Of course, the baby pulled at the sore, itching ears until she grabbed the hoops and subsequently tore her earlobes.

The newborn received two sutures to each lobe and we had a conversation with the mother about appropriate earrings for a baby.

--Z.P.
New York

Attempt

I worked as a counselor and aide in an assisted living facility. Our clients range between 18 and 55, and all our patients are mentally impaired, either because a birth defect or result of an accident.

I love and hate my career. I counsel patients when they feel hopeless or depressed. I also go back to my apartment and cry a lot. I've been in this position for thirty years and it hasn't gotten easier over time.

One patient who will forever hold a place in my heart is a woman who was suffering from postpartum depression. Her medication was not working, and her husband was unsupportive. The patient was left alone with her newborn and was responsible for the care of the couple's five-year-old, as well as responsible for keeping up the home and playing housewife.

The patient, while her oldest child was playing at the neighbor's house, decided to kill herself. She called her husband and left a message with his secretary, telling him to come home to take care of the baby and make sure their oldest child did not see her mother dead.

My patient did shoot herself, and a few moments later, her daughter and the child's friend walked inside. They ran back to the neighbor's house and the neighbor called 911. The patient's husband rushed home, but was too late to protect his daughter from viewing her mother's body.

This patient did not die. The bullet was lodged in her brain and she underwent surgery to remove it. She never fully recovered, neither mentally nor physically.

My patient spent her life waiting for her daughter to come home from the neighbor's house, and she almost always had a plastic baby doll in her arms. She had no idea that more than a decade had come to pass, and she didn't realize that her husband and daughters never came to visit because she was stuck in that time frame and never did know any different.

--Initials and location withheld at request

I responded to a call from a woman the morning after her one-night-stand.

She reported the man in her bed as deceased.

He was not deceased, he was just a heavy sleeper.

--D.M.
Oregon

Back to the Start

When I was five, my mother went into preterm labor. She called for help, but she hemorrhaged before an ambulance could arrive. Watching my mother die was the inspiration to become an emergency nurse. I did not want anyone to feel helpless in their time of desperation. I never wanted anyone to die alone.

All my life, I thought nursing would be spending every single day holding the hand of a dying patient. I thought I would smile with tears in my eyes as a patient thanked me for taking the time to listen when nobody else would. I imagined bringing relief to a patient in crippling pain. I imagined waving goodbye to a patient after he/she healed.

When I confided in my present-day coworkers about my hopes and dreams for my career, they admitted they once felt the same. We each have a story about why we entered the nursing field. Some of our stories are sadder than others. Nonetheless, we aim to offer superior care to our patients. We're not here for the paycheck. We're here for the patients, for the ailing, for the impaired, for the scared, for the hurting.

I learned quickly that my dreams of this career were so far off. Instead of holding hands, I find myself wiping butts and assisting drunk patients hold an emesis bag. I leave my shift covered in feces, blood, vomit, and semen—far from the picture-perfect shift ending I always imagined. Instead of grateful patients, I get the patients who scream, curse, and assault me because they had to wait three minutes, because I don't have pull over getting them a free cab, because the cafeteria is closed and no, they can't have a sandwich at three in the morning, when they come in stoned or drunk.

I sweat more than I thought I would. I cry more than I thought I would. I yawn more than I thought I would. I never dreamed of sore legs or feet so pained that I could hardly walk after a twelve-hour shift. I never planned on budgeting in compression socks or special-order gel inserts. When I was five, I didn't know my stethoscope would cost more than my car payment. I didn't imagine missing Thanksgiving, Christmas Eve, or my daughter's birthday because I was tending to someone presenting with a broken fingernail or diarrhea.

There are more days that I feel disposable than days I feel needed. Burnout rages through the emergency room on a normal basis and floors me quite often. I wake up after three hours of sleep and contemplate faking my death and moving to Argentina in order to avoid one more guiltless drunk driver or one more woman spitting on me because I tell her the doctor will not write her another prescription for the third bottle of pain meds 'stolen' this month.

What makes me feel fulfilled is performing CPR on a toddler. I feel needed when I'm doing chest compressions on an MVA victim. My heart is full when I pray with a woman who just learned she has a tumor in her lungs. I find my purpose all over again when I hug the mother of the 19-year-old man who just died from cerebral palsy.

Nursing is not easy, not on your body and not on your soul. I'm not sure there is any position involved with patients that is easy because you become involved with these people on a personal level, whether for five minutes or five days or five months. You see these patients and family members and friends at their most vulnerable. I've seen grown men fall to their knees in tears. I've seen frail old women hold it together for the sake of their grandchildren. In the ER, you see the side of others that they don't readily show the world, for good and bad.

Though there are many times I want to quit my job, I know I would never make it a month without nursing. I would probably hover around high-risk areas and wait for someone to keel over so I could help, because that is who I am.

I am a helper.

I am a hand holder.

I am a butt wiper, a patient flipper, and a colostomy bag changer.

I am a wife, a mother, and a charge nurse.

I am a crier. I am a laugher. I am someone who will wait with you while you're waiting for your son to arrive. I will call the nursing home for you if something does not seem 'right' about your care. I will spend hours on the phone with ten different charity organizations to help get you off the street or to help you pay for your prescriptions.

I know now that I will be disrespected again. I will go unappreciated by those with no compassion for others.

But I will never allow negativity to rub off on me. I will remain humble. I will remain compassionate. I will remain kind.

I am a nurse.

--T.K.
Indiana

A Message to Readers

Though I pushed for a few more pages, I thought the last submission was the best way to end this book. I am amazed at how selfless those in the medical field are. I strive to be that kind, dedicated, and compassionate.

Someone left a review that thanked me for enabling voice-reading for the Kindle. It brought me joy to know my books are being enjoyed by a vast range of readers. I value each of you, and I cannot thank you enough for being a fabulous audience. In case you are unaware or have forgotten, you may also find the audio version of '*A Double Dose of Dilaudid*' for purchase.

I'm sure you all know the drill here. If you have any comments, questions, or concerns, never hesitate to leave a review or send me a message/comment on a status. I will do my very best to respond quickly.

Have a great day!

Check me out on Twitter!

https://twitter.com/AuthorKerryHamm

My website:

http://www.authorkerryhamm.com

I'm also on Facebook. Drop a search for Author Kerry Hamm to find my page!

Printed in Great Britain
by Amazon